Secondary Procedures in Total Ankle Replacement

Editor

THOMAS S. ROUKIS

CLINICS IN PODIATRIC MEDICINE AND SURGERY

www.podiatric.theclinics.com

Consulting Editor
THOMAS ZGONIS

October 2015 • Volume 32 • Number 4

ELSEVIER

1600 John F. Kennedy Boulevard • Suite 1800 • Philadelphia, Pennsylvania, 19103-2899

http://www.theclinics.com

CLINICS IN PODIATRIC MEDICINE AND SURGERY Volume 32, Number 4
October 2015 ISSN 0891-8422, ISBN-13: 978-0-323-40102-9

Editor: Jennifer Flynn-Briggs
Developmental Editor: Alison Swety

Clinics in Podiatric Medicine and Surgery (ISSN 0891-8422) is published quarterly by Elsevier Inc., 360 Park Avenue South, New York, NY 10010-1710. Months of issue are January, April, July, and October. Business and Editorial Offices: 1600 John F. Kennedy Blvd., Ste. 1800, Philadelphia, PA 19103-2899. Customer Service Office: 3251 Riverport Lane, Maryland Heights, MO 63043. Periodicals postage paid at New York, NY and additional mailing offices. Subscription prices are $305.00 per year for US individuals, $450.00 per year for US institutions, $155.00 per year for US students and residents, $370.00 per year for Canadian individuals, $544.00 for Canadian institutions, $435.00 for international individuals, $544.00 per year for international institutions and $220.00 per year for Canadian and foreign students/residents. To receive student/resident rate, orders must be accompanied by name of affiliated institution, date of term, and the *signature* of program/residency coordinator on institution letterhead. Orders will be billed at individual rate until proof of status is received. Foreign air speed delivery is included in all *Clinics* subscription prices. All prices are subject to change without notice. POSTMASTER: Send address changes to *Clinics in Podiatric Medicine and Surgery*, Elsevier Health Sciences Division, Subscription Customer Service, 3251 Riverport Lane, Maryland Heights, MO 63043. **Customer Service: 1-800-654-2452 (US). From outside of the US, call 314-447-8871. Fax: 314-447-8029. E-mail: JournalsCustomerService-usa@elsevier.com (for print support); JournalsOnlineSupport-usa@elsevier.com (for online support).**

Reprints. For copies of 100 or more of articles in this publication, please contact the Commercial Reprints Department, Elsevier Inc., 360 Park Avenue South, New York, NY 10010-1710. Tel.: 212-633-3874; Fax: 212-633-3820; E-mail: reprints@elsevier.com.

Clinics in Podiatric Medicine and Surgery is covered in *MEDLINE/PubMed (Index Medicus) and EMBASE/Excerpta Medica.*

CLINICS IN PODIATRIC MEDICINE AND SURGERY

CONSULTING EDITOR
THOMAS ZGONIS, DPM, FACFAS

Contributors

CONSULTING EDITOR

THOMAS ZGONIS, DPM, FACFAS
Professor and Director, Externship and Reconstructive Foot and Ankle Fellowship
Programs, Division of Podiatric Medicine and Surgery, Department of Orthopedics,
University of Texas Health Science Center San Antonio, San Antonio, Texas

EDITOR

THOMAS S. ROUKIS, DPM, PhD, FACFAS
Orthopaedic Center, Gundersen Health System, La Crosse, Wisconsin

AUTHORS

ANNETTE F.P. BARTEL, DPM, MPH
Podiatric Medicine and Surgery Resident (PGY-III), Gundersen Medical Foundation,
La Crosse, Wisconsin

THOMAS C. BEIDEMAN, DPM
Chief Podiatric Surgery Resident, Mercy Suburban Hospital, Norristown, Pennsylvania

ANDREW D. ELLIOTT, DPM, JD
Podiatric Medicine and Surgery Resident (PGY-III), Gundersen Medical Foundation,
La Crosse, Wisconsin

NIKOLAOS GOUGOULIAS, MD, PhD
Department of Trauma and Orthopaedics, Frimley Health NHS Foundation Trust, Frimley
Park Hospital, Surrey, United Kingdom

TUN HING LUI, MBBS (HK), FRCS (Edin), FHKAM, FHKCOS
Consultant, Department of Orthopaedics and Traumatology, North District Hospital, Hong
Kong SAR, China

NICOLA MAFFULLI, MD, MS, PhD, FRCP, FRCS (Orth)
Department of Musculoskeletal Disorders, Faculty of Medicine and Surgery, University of
Salerno, Salerno, Italy; Centre for Sports and Exercise Medicine, Barts and The London
School of Medicine and Dentistry, Mile End Hospital, London, United Kingdom

BENJAMIN D. OVERLEY Jr, DPM, FACFAS
Foot and Ankle Specialist, PMSI Division of Orthopedics, Pottstown, Pennsylvania

THOMAS S. ROUKIS, DPM, PhD, FACFAS
Orthopaedic Center, Gundersen Health System, La Crosse, Wisconsin

DEVIN C. SIMONSON, DPM, AACFAS
Orthopaedic Center, Gundersen Health System, La Crosse, Wisconsin

Contents

Surgeons performing primary total ankle replacement have achieved outcomes comparable to ankle arthrodesis. However, while many reports exist suggesting the presence of a surgeon learning curve period during initial performance of primary total ankle replacement, no published analysis of the actual incidence of complications encountered during this period exists. Therefore, we sought to provide such an analysis through systematic review. A total of 2453 primary total ankle replacements with 1085 complications (44.2%) were identified. Our results revealed conflicting data whether an acceptably low incidence of high-grade complications leading to total ankle replacement failure exists during the surgeon learning curve period.

National joint registry data provides unique information about primary total ankle replacement (TAR) survival. We sought to recreate survival curves among published national joint registry data sets using the Kaplan-Meier estimator. Overall, 5152 primary and 591 TAR revisions were included over a 2- to 13-year period with prosthesis survival for all national joint registries of 0.94 at 2-years, 0.87 at 5-years and 0.81 at 10-years. National joint registry datasets should strive for completion of data presentation including revision definitions, modes and time of failure, and patients lost to follow-up or death for complete accuracy of the Kaplan-Meier estimator.

There is great potential of managing the complications of total ankle replacement arthroscopically and endoscopically, and these procedures can be summarized into 3 groups. Group 1 includes procedures of the ankle joint proper with close proximity to the articular components of the total ankle replacement. Group 2 includes procedures of the tibia and talus with close proximity to the nonarticular parts of the total ankle replacement. Group 3 includes procedures that are away from the total ankle replacement. However, these remain master arthroscopist procedures and should be performed by foot and ankle surgeons who perform them with regularity.

The development of osteophytes, ectopic bone, or malleolar impingement following total ankle replacement represents common complications that will frequently lead to secondary procedures to relieve painful impingement. Many studies have been conducted to discover the cause of these postoperative impingement syndromes; however, there is a paucity of literature with regard to the prevention, diagnosis, and management of these conditions. The authors discuss the potential causes of formation of osteophytes and ectopic bone formation, as well as malleolar impingement syndromes following primary total ankle replacement with focus placed on diagnosis and management of these complications.

Achieving frontal plane alignment of the ankle joint during total ankle replacement is essential for long-term success. Tendon and ligament lengthening, ligament reinforcement, tendon transfer, nonanatomic tendon transfer ligament reconstruction, and periarticular osteotomies are safe, straightforward, minimally invasive, and reproducible procedures to correct varus and valgus deformities associated with end-stage degenerative joint disease. Using reproducible topographic anatomic landmarks is essential to perform these techniques properly and limit complications. The approach to frontal plane deformities is stepwise, with liberal use of tendon and ligament lengthening and reconstruction, a low threshold for nonanatomic tendon transfer ligament reconstructions, and tendon transfers and/or periarticular osteotomies.

Total ankle replacement remains an option for varus and valgus ankles, provided that it results in a balanced, neutrally aligned ankle. Accurate preoperative assessment of the deformity is essential for appropriate selection of adjuvant procedures. Osteotomies performed proximal (tibial), within (malleolar), or distal to (calcaneal, metatarsal) the ankle, allow deformity correction. Outcomes can be expected to be as good as of those ankles without coronal plane malalignment, at least in the short-term.

Management of Osseous and Soft-Tissue Ankle Equinus During Total Ankle Replacement   543

Thomas S. Roukis and Devin C. Simonson

Obtaining functional alignment of a total ankle replacement, including physiologic sagittal plane range of motion, is paramount for a successful outcome. This article reviews the literature on techniques available for correction of osseous and soft-tissue equinus at the time of index total ankle replacement. These techniques include anterior tibiotalar joint cheilectomy, posterior superficial muscle compartment lengthening, posterior ankle capsule release, and release of the posterior portions of the medial and lateral collateral ligament complexes. The rationale for these procedures and the operative sequence of events for these procedures are presented.

The Salto Talaris XT Revision Ankle Prosthesis   551

Thomas S. Roukis

The Salto Talaris XT Revision Ankle Prosthesis is an anatomically designed fixed-bearing prosthesis available in the United States based on the design of previous Salto systems. The Salto Talaris XT Revision Ankle Prosthesis design optimizes surface area, cortical contact, and ultrahigh-molecular-weight polyethylene conformity. Two tibial component designs, both with the same base plate dimensions, are available, the standard conical fixation plug affixed to a short keel and a long-stemmed version. The author presents an overview of the Salto Talaris XT Revision Ankle Prosthesis surgical technique and pearls for successful application.

Incidence of Complications During Initial Experience with Revision of the Agility and Agility LP Total Ankle Replacement Systems: A Single Surgeon's Learning Curve Experience   569

Thomas S. Roukis and Devin C. Simonson

As the frequency in which foot and ankle surgeons are performing primary total ankle replacement (TAR) continues to build, revision TAR will likely become more commonplace, creating a need for an established benchmark by which to evaluate the safety of revision TAR as determined by the incidence of complications. Currently, no published data exist on the incidence of intraoperative and early postoperative complications during revision of the Agility or Agility LP Total Ankle Replacement Systems during the surgeon learning curve period; therefore, the authors sought to determine this incidence during the senior author's learning curve period.

Management of Massive Hindfoot Osteolysis Secondary to Failed INBONE I Total Ankle Replacement   595

Thomas S. Roukis

This article presents a procedure whereby a failed INBONE I saddle talar component and polyethylene insert associated with massive cystic changes within the talus and calcaneus secondary to aseptic osteolysis was treated with impaction cancellous allograft bone graft impregnated with autogenous proximal tibia bone marrow aspirate and conversion to an INBONE II sulcus talar component and polyethylene insert. Concomitantly, a percutaneous tendo-Achilles lengthening and posterior capsule release was performed to enhance ankle dorsiflexion. The rationale for these procedures, the operative sequence of events, and recovery course are presented in detail. Causes for concern regarding subsequent revision, should this be required, are raised.

This article presents a rare case involving combined revision of a failed Agility Total Ankle Replacement System (DePuy Orthopaedics, Warsaw, Indiana) and open reduction with internal fixation of periprosthetic midfoot fractures secondary to acute traumatic injury. The rationale for these procedures, the operative sequence of events, and recovery course are presented in detail. Causes for concern regarding subsequent revision, should this be required, are raised.

CLINICS IN PODIATRIC MEDICINE AND SURGERY

RELATED INTEREST

Foot and Ankle Clinics, March 2015 (Vol. 20, Issue 1)
Arthroscopy and Endoscopy
Rebecca A. Cerrato, *Editor*
Available at: http://www.foot.theclinics.com/

THE CLINICS ARE AVAILABLE ONLINE!
Access your subscription at:
www.theclinics.com

RELATED INTEREST

Foreword

Secondary Procedures in Total Ankle Replacement

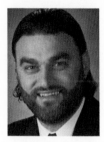

Thomas Zgonis, DPM, FACFAS
Consulting Editor

This issue of *Clinics in Podiatric Medicine and Surgery* is focused on secondary procedures in Total Ankle Replacement (TAR) and is completing previous issues on primary and revisional TAR led by our guest editor, Dr Roukis. Secondary procedures in TAR include a wide variety of surgical entities including but not limited to periarticular foot and ankle osteotomies, tendinous/ligamentous reconstruction, and arthrodesis of adjacent joints.

From a systemic review of complications during the surgeon's learning curve on primary TAR to arthroscopic management and osteotomies addressing lower extremity deformities along with TAR, this issue of *Clinics in Podiatric Medicine and Surgery* complements our series on TAR available in the United States. Great emphasis is given to the detailed preoperative planning and technological advances in TAR with special attention to deformity correction that might be addressed in a staged reconstruction.

Finally, I would like to thank the guest editor, invited authors, and our readers for their continuous support of *Clinics in Podiatric Medicine and Surgery*.

Thomas Zgonis, DPM, FACFAS
Externship and Reconstructive Foot & Ankle Fellowship Programs
Division of Podiatric Medicine and Surgery
Department of Orthopedics
University of Texas Health Science Center San Antonio
7703 Floyd Curl Drive–MSC 7776
San Antonio, TX 78229, USA

E-mail address:
zgonis@uthscsa.edu

Clin Podiatr Med Surg 32 (2015) xiii
http://dx.doi.org/10.1016/j.cpm.2015.07.005
0891-8422/15/$ – see front matter © 2015 Published by Elsevier Inc.

podiatric.theclinics.com

Preface

Secondary Procedures in Total Ankle Replacement

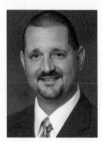

Thomas S. Roukis, DPM, PhD, FACFAS
Editor

It is with great pleasure that I serve as guest editor for this issue of *Clinics in Podiatric Medicine and Surgery* devoted to Secondary Procedures in Total Ankle Replacement, which is the final follow-up issue to Primary Total Ankle Replacement, published in January 2013, and Revision Total Ankle Replacement, published in April 2013.

The definition of secondary procedures includes nonrevisional surgery following primary implantation of total ankle replacement involving the joint (ie, termed reoperation and includes debridement, incidental polyethylene insert exchange, or wound treatment) or not involving the joint (ie, termed additional procedures and includes ligament reconstruction/release, adjacent joint arthrodesis, adjacent periarticular osteotomy, or tendon lengthening/transfer). This is to differentiate these secondary procedures from formal revision surgery defined as failure of the total ankle replacement system components sufficient to warrant manipulation and/or removal of the tibial and/or talar components with reimplantation using an alternative system or custom-designed implants; conversion to an arthrodesis; or amputation of the limb. Whenever possible, the focus through the issue is on total ankle replacement systems available for use in the United States.

We start this *Clinics in Podiatric Medicine and Surgery* issue with a systematic review of the literature for complications encountered during primary total ankle replacement, followed by an analysis of registry data regarding complications with primary total ankle replacement. We then focus on management of postoperative stiffness, soft tissue impingement, painful osteophytes, osseous impingement, and pain in the malleolar gutters. Management of varus and valgus malalignment utilizing tendon transfers and osteotomies as well as management of osseous and soft tissue equinus with total ankle replacement follows. We then review the Salto Talaris XT Revision Ankle Prosthesis (Tornier, Inc, Bloomington, MN, USA) intended for use when secondary procedures are not appropriate and conversion of a failed total ankle replacement is required. This is followed by reviewing the incidence of complications encountered

Clin Podiatr Med Surg 32 (2015) xv–xvi
http://dx.doi.org/10.1016/j.cpm.2015.07.004
0891-8422/15/$ – see front matter © 2015 Published by Elsevier Inc.

podiatric.theclinics.com

during a single surgeon's learning curve experience with revision of the Agility and Agility LP Total Ankle Replacement Systems (DePuy Synthes Joint Reconstruction, Warsaw, IN, USA). We conclude by reviewing interesting cases involving the management of failed total ankle replacement following massive hindfoot osteolysis and acute traumatic periprosthetic fracture.

The intent of this issue is to provide up-to-date information available for the challenging problems associated with secondary surgery following total ankle replacement. It is hoped that the readers of this issue of *Clinics in Podiatric Medicine and Surgery* will enjoy these articles as much as I have.

Thomas S. Roukis, DPM, PhD, FACFAS
Orthopaedic Center
Gundersen Health System
Mail Stop: CO2-006
1900 South Avenue
La Crosse, WI 54601-5467, USA

E-mail address:
tsroukis@gundersenhealth.org

Incidence of Complications During the Surgeon Learning Curve Period for Primary Total Ankle Replacement

A Systematic Review

Devin C. Simonson, DPM, Thomas S. Roukis, DPM, PhD*

KEYWORDS

• Arthroplasty • Complications • Prosthesis • Tibiotalar joint • Surgery

KEY POINTS

- Advances in technology for total ankle replacement have renewed the popularity of this procedure as an alternative to ankle arthrodesis.
- A systematic review of the world literature reveals that the overall incidence of complications encountered during the surgeons' learning curve period for primary total ankle replacement, regardless of prosthesis system, is 44.2% (1085 of 2453).
- The rate of a complication progressing to failure carries more clinical importance than the general incidence of any complication.
- A comparison of 2 classification systems reveals conflicting data as to whether an acceptably low incidence of high-grade complications leading to ultimate total ankle replacement failure exists during the surgeon learning curve period.
- A validated classification system is needed to allow more standardized reporting of complications encountered in the surgeon learning curve period for primary total ankle replacement.

INTRODUCTION

The emergence, initial failure, and subsequent resurgence of total ankle replacement (TAR) as a viable alternative to ankle arthrodesis for the treatment of end-stage ankle arthritis is well documented.[1–8] Improved surgeon training and usage of current-generation TAR systems have produced better patient outcomes.[1–13] As a result,

Financial Disclosure: None.

Conflicts of Interest: None.

Orthopaedic Center, Gundersen Health System, Mail Stop: CO2-006, 1900 South Avenue, La Crosse, WI 54601, USA

* Corresponding author.

E-mail address: tsroukis@gundersenhealth.org

foot and ankle surgeons competent in primary TAR have now achieved outcomes comparable with, if not superior to, ankle arthrodesis[1–3,11]; however, there is a learning curve for surgeons during their initial use of various TAR systems.[1–10,12] As clinicians progress further into the reality of primary TAR being more routinely performed, revision TAR will also continue to become more common. It is reasonable to assume that most complications leading to revision will occur during the surgeons' learning curve period of primary TAR. However, although many reports suggest the presence of a learning curve, there is no published analysis of the exact incidence of complications encountered during the surgeons' learning curve period for primary TAR, regardless of prosthesis system. This article provides such an analysis, in order to establish data by which patients and surgeons alike can expect to encounter the various complications specific to primary TAR during the surgeons' learning curve period. Furthermore, it is hoped that this may then afford surgeons a benchmark by which to compare the safety of primary and revision TAR during their learning curve period.

MATERIALS AND METHODS

We used the PRISMA (Preferred Reporting Items for Systematic Reviews and Meta-analyses) guidelines.[14] Accordingly, electronic databases and relevant peer-reviewed sources including OvidSP/MEDLINE (http://ovidsp.tx.ovid.com) and PubMed (http://www.ncbi.nlm.nih.gov/pubmed/) were searched from inception to August 2014 with no restriction on date or language, and using an inclusive text word query "ankle" AND "replacement" OR "arthroplasty" OR "implant" OR "prosthesis" AND "learning curve" in which the uppercase words represent the Boolean operators used. Only articles that specifically reported a surgeon's initial patient cohort undergoing primary TAR, regardless of system, and that included all complications encountered during this learning curve period were considered. The references from the identified studies were individually searched for additional potentially pertinent published works, which were then obtained for review. We also manually searched common American, British, and European orthopedic and podiatric scientific literature for relevant articles. In addition, by using various combinations of the text words listed earlier, an Internet-based scholarly literature search engine, specifically Google Scholar (http://scholar.google.com/; last accessed August 8, 2014) was used to identify available sources that could potentially provide useful information.

Both authors reviewed all the articles and complete agreement was necessary for final inclusion, with the lead author being the moderator. Only full-text, published articles were considered. No reports were excluded based on an inability to obtain them. If the reference was not written in English, the contents of the reference were translated from its native language of French or German to English using an Internet-based translator (Google Translate; available at: http://translate.google.com/#; last accessed August 8, 2014).

In addition, the level of evidence of each individual study was determined according to the evidence-based medicine grading system recommended by the American College of Foot and Ankle Surgeons (http://www.jfas.org/authorinfo; last accessed August 8, 2014).

RESULTS

The search for potentially eligible information for inclusion in the systematic review yielded a total of 351 articles. After considering all the potentially eligible articles, 25 (7.1%) studies met our inclusion criteria (**Fig. 1**), involving a total of 2453 TARs (2414 patients) and 12 different TAR systems (**Table 1**). In the studies that included

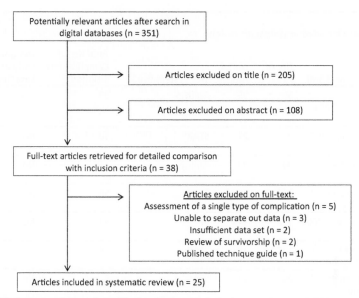

Fig. 1. The reports during the selection process.

gender, there were 1142 (51.6%) women and 1070 (48.4%) men. The weighted mean age of the patients was 59.8 years (range, 18–89 years) and the weighted mean follow-up was 29.3 months (range, 1.5–240 months). The reported indication for primary TAR was most commonly posttraumatic arthritis (50.9%) followed by primary end-stage arthritis (25.6%), rheumatoid arthritis (16.5%), and "other" (5.8%), which included various inflammatory arthritides, pseudarthrosis following attempted arthrodesis, and hemochromatosis. The indication was not specified in 1.2% of cases. There were a total of 1090 complications reported during the surgeon learning curve period; however, of these, 5 involved deep vein thrombosis and were excluded because this complication is germane to all surgery. Therefore, we identified 1085 complications, yielding an overall incidence of complications of 44.2% (1085 of 2453).

The incidence of complications was 60.8% (141 of 232) for the Agility TAR system (DePuy Orthopaedics, Warsaw, IN); 51.9% (82 of 158) for the Hintegra Total Ankle Prosthesis (Integra, Saint Priest, France); 47.9% (650 of 1356) for the Scandinavian TAR system (STAR, Waldemar Link, Hamburg, Germany/Small Bone Innovations, Inc, Morrisville, PA/Stryker Orthopaedics, Mahwah, NJ); 29.7% (41 of 138) for the Ankle Evolutive System (AES, Transystème–JMT Implants, Nimes, France); 24.1% (14 of 58) for the INBONE I TAR (Wright Medical Technology, Inc, Memphis, TN); 23.3% (14 of 60) for the Salto Mobile Version Prosthesis (Tornier NV, Amsterdam, The Netherlands); 21.7% (13 of 60) for the Mobility Total Ankle System (DePuy, Leeds, United Kingdom); and 14.9% (10 of 67) for the Salto Talaris Total Ankle Prosthesis (Tornier, Inc, Bloomington, MN). The incidence of complications for the remaining 209 prostheses was 29.2% (61 of 209) but could not be separated out by the specific TAR systems. Only 24% (6 of 25) of the publications, involving 990 TAR prostheses, designated the complications as occurring either early or late. The incidence of complications in these studies was 54.9% (543 of 990).

The methodological quality of the included studies was generally fair. For the studies involving complications encountered during the surgeon learning curve period for primary TAR, regardless of specific system, all were full-text articles. One study

Table 1
Study data included in systematic review

Author, Year (EBM)	No. of Patients	No. of Ankles	TAR System (No.)	Total No. of Complications Included	Designated Early and Late Groups?
Myerson & Mroczek,[4] 2003 (IV)	50	50	Agility[a]	39	Yes
Natens et al,[5] 2003 (IV)	25	27	STAR[b]	10	No
Saltzman et al,[15] 2003 (IV)	90	90	Agility	41	No
Wood & Deakin,[16] 2003 (IV)	200	200	STAR	90	No
Buechel et al,[17] 2004 (IV)	112	115	BP[c]	59	No
Haskell & Mann,[18] 2004 (IV)	187	187	STAR	79	Yes
Murnaghan et al,[6] 2005 (IV)	20	22	STAR	9	No
Schuberth et al,[7] 2006 (IV)	48	50	Agility	51	No
Harris et al,[19] 2007 (IV)	138	138	AES[d]	41	No
Kumar & Dhar,[8] 2007 (IV)	43	50	STAR	27	Yes
Álvarez-Goenaga,[20] 2008 (IV)	25	25	Hintegra[e]	18	No
Lee et al,[21] 2008 (III)	50	50	Hintegra	32	Yes
Saltzman et al,[2] 2009 (II)	593	593	STAR	353	Yes
Bai et al,[22] 2010 (III)	65	67	Hintegra	26	No
Reuver et al,[9] 2010 (IV)	55	60	Salto[f]	14	No
Criswell et al,[23] 2012 (IV)	41	42	Agility	10	No
Pinar et al,[24] 2012 (IV)	179	183	Salto (91), Hintegra (39), AES (20), Coppélia[g] (17), STAR (11), Ramses[h] (4), Akilé CLL[i] (1)	52	No
Bleazey et al,[10] 2013 (IV)	57	58	INBONE[j]	14	No
Brunner et al,[25] 2013 (IV)	72	77	STAR	12	No
Clement et al,[1] 2013 (IV)	24	26	STAR (14), Salto Talaris[k] (11), INBONE (1)	9	No
Lee et al,[26] 2013 (III)	60	60	Mobility[l]	13	Yes

(continued on next page)

Table 1 (continued)					
Author, Year (EBM)	No. of Patients	No. of Ankles	TAR System (No.)	Total No. of Complications Included	Designated Early and Late Groups?
Noelle et al,[11] 2013 (IV)	97	100	STAR	22	No
Schimmel et al,[12] 2013 (IV)	100	100	STAR	48	No
Schweitzer et al,[27] 2013 (IV)	67	67	Salto Talaris	10	No
Willegger et al,[13] 2013 (IV)	16	16	Hintegra	6	No
Total	2414	2453	—	1085	6 Yes/19 No

Abbreviations: EBM, evidence-based medicine; No., number.
  [a] Agility TAR (DePuy Orthopaedics, Inc, Warsaw, IN).
  [b] Scandinavian TAR (LINK STAR, Waldemar Link, Hamburg, Germany/Small Bone Innovations, Inc, Morrisville, PA/Stryker Orthopaedics, Mahwah, NJ).
  [c] Buechel-Pappas (BP, Endotec, South Orange, NJ).
  [d] AES (Transystème-JMT Implants, Nimes, France).
  [e] Hintegra Total Ankle Prosthesis (Integra, Saint Priest, France).
  [f] Salto Mobile Version Ankle Prosthesis (Tornier, Saint-Martin, France).
  [g] Coppélia (Unknown Manufacturer, France).
  [h] Ramses Ankle Replacement (Laboratoire Fournitures Hospitalières Industrie, Heimsbrunn, France).
  [i] Akilé CLL (Centre Hospitalier Universitaire de Bordeux, Bordeux, France).
  [j] INBONE I TAR (Wright Medical Technology, Inc, Memphis, TN).
  [k] Salto Talaris Total Ankle Prosthesis (Tornier, Edina, MN).
  [l] Mobility Total Ankle System (DePuy UK, Leeds, England).

was considered evidence-based medicine (EBM) level II, 3 studies were EBM level III, and the remaining 21 were EBM level IV studies, as identified in Table 1.[1,2,4–8,10–13,15–27] All studies were published in known peer-reviewed journals.

DISCUSSION

The purpose of this systematic review was to determine the incidence of complications encountered during the surgeon learning curve period for the initial performance of primary TAR, regardless of specific prosthesis system used. Our review identified 1085 reported complications, yielding an incidence of complications encountered during the surgeon learning curve period for primary TAR of 44.2%. Taken as a whole, the highly variable severity, long-term consequences of the numerous encountered complications, and variability of specific TAR used greatly devalue the discovered incidence; therefore we decided to further extrapolate these data so as to be more useful to patients considering, and surgeons performing, primary TAR.

In 2009, Glazebrook and colleagues[28] proposed a classification system based on the rate of failure for a given complication encountered during primary TAR published in the literature. Although the investigators admitted that the clinical significance of their classification system was questionable because the reliability had yet to be investigated at the time of publication, they found 3 categories of complications correlating with the likelihood of the complication leading to failure of primary TAR. These categories were low, medium, and high grade, which were described respectively as being very unlikely to cause TAR failure, leading to failure less than 50% of the time, or leading to failure greater than or equal to 50% of the time. Low-grade complications included intraoperative bone fracture and wound healing problems; medium-grade complications included technical error, subsidence, and postoperative bone fracture; and high-grade complications included deep infection, aseptic loosening, and prosthesis failure. We agree with the investigators that the rate of a complication progressing to failure carries more clinical importance than the general incidence of any complication because it serves as a better indicator of the severity of a particular complication.

Based on our collection of reported data, we were able to categorize nearly all complications as described by Glazebrook and colleagues.[28] Out of the reported 1085 complications, 112 (10.3%) were considered high grade, 209 (19.3%) were medium grade, 588 (54.2%) were low grade, and 176 (16.2%) were unclassified. The unclassified complications included nerve and tendon injuries, and could be considered technical error, thus classifying them as medium-grade complications; however, these specific injuries are not explicitly defined in their article. Presented from a different perspective, based on the number of complications encountered from the entire cohort included in our data, a foot and ankle surgeon new to primary TAR could reasonably expect the overall incidence of high-grade, medium-grade, and low-grade complications encountered during the initial learning curve period for primary TAR to be 4.6% (112 of 2453), 8.5% (209 of 2453), and 24% (588 of 2453) respectively, and the incidence of encountering an unclassified complication (specifically nerve or tendon injury) to be 7.1% (176 of 2453).

Recently, Gadd and colleagues[29] investigated the reliability of the literature-based classification system proposed by Glazebrook and colleagues,[28] based on their tertiary referral center in the United Kingdom. Their published data of 212 primary TARs revealed an incidence of revision of 17% (n = 36). Every complication aside from intraoperative bone fracture and wound healing problems led to prosthesis failure greater than or equal to 50% of the time. Based on their data, they proposed a simplification of the Glazebrook and colleagues[28] classification system by which only 2 grades of complications exist: high and low. Because both intraoperative bone fracture and wound healing problems are unlikely to lead to implant failure, these would constitute low-grade complications. All other potential complications would then be classified as high grade, meaning they have a greater than or equal to 50% incidence of failure. Gadd and colleagues[29] agreed that a validated classification system would improve consistency in reporting primary TAR complications; however, they found the proposed 3-tiered system by Glazebrook and colleagues[28] to be unreliable. We agree with Gadd and colleagues[29] that timely recognition and treatment of all complications is imperative, because this decreases the likelihood of primary TAR failure and poor clinical outcome.

Based on the Gadd and colleagues[29] classification, out of the reported 1085 complications identified in our systematic review, 321 (29.6%) were considered high grade, 576 (54.2%) were low grade, and 176 (16.2%) were unclassified, which again included nerve and tendon injuries. The results from categorizing complications using the 2-tiered system by Gadd and colleagues[29] suggests nearly a 3-fold increase in the incidence of complications leading to implant failure compared with the results when categorized using the 3-tiered system by Glazebrook and colleagues.[28]

Numerous weaknesses of this study were considered. First, as a result of the electronic searches included, it is possible that pertinent references were inadvertently excluded or overlooked. However, the inclusion criteria were intentionally defined in broad terms so that as many references as possible could be included and bias would be reduced. Similarly, because we limited our search to only certain languages we may have induced bias toward accepting articles published in English, French, and German speaking countries. However, our exhaustive search electronically was further supplemented by individually searching all references and major medical journals germane to research published on TAR. With such a detailed search, it is unlikely that pertinent references that would alter the investigators' conclusions were overlooked. The inclusion of only published articles may have induced bias into our conclusions because studies with poorer outcomes may have elected not to publish their data after presenting it at a congress or similar event. However, we have no way of controlling for this. Another potential weakness involves a discrepancy in the overall investigator experience in the included studies, with some investigators being established foot and ankle surgeons with no prior primary TAR experience, whereas other surgeons had prior, and at times even extensive, primary TAR experience but were reporting on a new or unfamiliar primary TAR system. Although this provides heterogeneity among the reviewed articles, the overall incidence of complications encountered during the surgeon learning curve period, regardless of TAR system, was the primary objective of this systematic review. Another weakness includes the possible inflation of the overall incidence of complications based on studies not specifically indicating whether a given patient experienced multiple complications. In addition, we could not account for the assumed abbreviated learning curve period of current-generation TAR systems as opposed to older generations that likely involved a higher incidence of various complications during the surgeon learning curve period. Note that complications identified for the Agility TAR (60.8%), Hintegra Total Ankle Prosthesis (51.9%), and STAR (47.1%) were 2 to 4 times as frequent as complications for the AES (29.7%), INBONE I TAR (24.1%), Salto Mobile Version Ankle Prosthesis (23.3%), Mobility Total Ankle System (21.7%), and Salto Talaris Total Ankle Prosthesis (14.9%). However, the significance of this remains unknown because the first grouping consisted of multiple studies and a much larger number of primary TARs, whereas the second grouping included only isolated studies and a small number of primary TARs. Note that, although we found reports of 12 different prosthesis systems, our review is not all-encompassing and other TAR prostheses are available and routinely implanted. For example, we found an unpublished case series that reported on the initial 45 TAR procedures performed by a single surgeon using the Zimmer Trabecular Metal TAR (Herbst S, Current Zimmer Series SAH: Learning Curve Data, presented via the Zimmer Trabecular Meta TAR Patient Outcomes & Interactive Case Review Webinar; https://zio.zimmer.com/learncenter.asp, last accessed July 13, 2014). The author's data revealed a total of 11 complications, for an overall incidence of complications of 24.4% (11 of 45). None of the reported complications would have been classified as high grade under the Glazebrook and colleagues[28] classification system; however, according to the Gadd and colleagues[29] classification system, all 11 complications would be considered high grade. Although these data did not meet our inclusion criteria, we discuss them here simply to further show the paucity of and need for continued research into the surgeon learning curve period for all TAR prostheses. This single unpublished data set clearly shows the need for a validated classification system to allow more standardized reporting of complications encountered during the surgeon learning curve period for their initial performance of primary TAR. Similarly, the impact of intramedullary versus extramedullary referencing,[30] computer-assisted bone preparation,[31] and computed tomography (CT) scan–derived patient-specific guides[32–34] on the surgeon learning curve period during initial performance of primary TAR remain unknown and warrant further investigation. Another weakness is in the reporting of complications encountered within the surgeon learning curve period. Many studies mentioned the presence of a surgeon learning curve period; however, few studies presented separate patient cohorts for early and late groups in order to identify trends in their incidence of complications over time. Many studies simply reported on the first group of patients undergoing primary TAR with a particular prosthesis system, and anecdotally identified a reduced incidence of complications over time. Specifically, the timing of complication occurrence as either early or late was reported for only 40% (990 of 2453) of the TARs performed involving 50% (543 of 1085) of the complications reported. If more studies existed that clearly identified all complications encountered in distinct groups (ie, early vs late) in the surgeons' learning curve period, the strength of our review would be improved. In addition, we did not evaluate for the effect that selection (inventor) or publication (conflict of interest) bias may have had on the incidence of complications encountered during the surgeon learning curve period. As a result, the incidence of complications may be higher than the rate we identified in our systematic review. However, the true effect, if any, that selection or bias may have had on the incidence of complications encountered during the surgeon learning curve period remains unanswered.

In conclusion, we performed a systematic review using electronic databases to determine the incidence of complications encountered during the surgeon learning curve period for primary TAR, regardless of prosthesis system used. Based on the inclusion criteria, a total of 25 studies involving 12 different TAR systems were included in the analysis. The overall incidence of complications was 44.2% during the surgeon learning curve period for primary TAR irrespective of the specific prosthesis system used. These complications were categorically divided based on the classification system proposed by Glazebrook and colleagues[28] as well as the simplified system proposed by Gadd and colleagues.[29] Under the Glazebrook and colleagues[28] classification system, 10.3% were considered high grade, 19.3% medium grade, and 54.2% low grade. Under the Gadd and colleagues[29] classification system, 29.6% were considered high grade and 54.2% were low grade. According to each classification system, the incidence of unclassified complications was 16.2%. Based on these findings, there are conflicting data as to whether an acceptably low incidence of high-grade complications exists in the surgeon learning curve period for primary TAR, regardless of prosthetic system used. A validated classification system is needed to allow more standardized reporting of complications encountered during the surgeon learning curve period. In addition, more studies analyzing a separation of patient cohorts into early and late groups would allow the duration of the surgeon learning curve period to be accurately defined. Moreover, comparison of complications encountered with primary implantation of current-generation fixed-bearing and mobile-bearing TAR systems during the surgeon learning curve period, as well as the impact of intramedullary versus extramedullary referencing, computer-assisted bone preparation, and CT scan–derived patient-specific guides, all warrant further investigation.

REFERENCES

1. Clement RC, Krynetskiy E, Parekh SG. The total ankle arthroplasty learning curve with third-generation implants. Foot Ankle Spec 2013;6:263–70.
2. Saltzman CL, Mann RA, Ahrens JE, et al. Prospective controlled trial of STAR total ankle replacement versus ankle fusion: initial results. Foot Ankle Int 2009;30: 579–96.
3. Esparragoza L, Vidal C, Vaquero J. Comparative study of the quality of life between arthrodesis and total arthroplasty substitution of the ankle. J Foot Ankle Surg 2011;50:383–7.

4. Myerson MS, Mroczek K. Perioperative complications of total ankle arthroplasty. Foot Ankle Int 2003;24:17–21.

5. Natens P, Dereymaeker G, Abbara M, et al. Early results after four years experience with the STAR uncemented total ankle prosthesis. Acta Orthop Belg 2003; 69:49–58.

6. Murnaghan JM, Warnock DS, Henderson SA. Total ankle replacement. Early experiences with STAR prosthesis. Ulster Med J 2005;74:9–13.

7. Schuberth JM, Patel S, Zarutsky E. Perioperative complications of the Agility total ankle replacement in 50 initial, consecutive cases. J Foot Ankle Surg 2006;45: 139–46.

8. Kumar A, Dhar S. Total ankle replacement: early results during learning period. Foot Ankle Surg 2007;13:19–23.

9. Reuver JM, Dayerizadeh N, Burger B, et al. Total ankle replacement outcome in low volume centers: short-term follow-up. Foot Ankle Int 2010;31:1064–8.

10. Bleazey ST, Brigido SA, Protzman NM. Perioperative complications of a modular stem fixed-bearing total ankle replacement with intramedullary guidance. J Foot Ankle Surg 2013;52:36–41.

11. Noelle S, Egidy CC, Cross MB, et al. Complication rates after total ankle arthroplasty in one hundred consecutive prostheses. Int Orthop 2013;37:1789–94.

12. Schimmel JJ, Walschot LH, Louwerens JW. Comparison of the short-term results of the first and last 50 Scandinavian Total Ankle Replacements: assessment of the learning curve in a consecutive series. Foot Ankle Int 2013;35:326–33.

13. Willegger M, Trnka HJ, Schuh R. The Hintegra ankle arthroplasty: intermediate term results of 16 consecutive ankles and a review on the current literature. Clin Res Foot Ankle 2013;2:124.

14. Liberati A, Altman DG, Tetzlaff J, et al. The PRISMA statement for reporting systematic reviews and meta-analyses of studies that evaluate health care interventions: explanation and elaboration. Ann Intern Med 2009;151:65–94.

15. Saltzman CL, Amendola A, Anderson R, et al. Surgeon training and complications in total ankle arthroplasty. Foot Ankle Int 2003;24:514–8.

16. Wood PL, Deakin S. Total ankle replacement: the results in 200 ankles. J Bone Joint Surg Br 2003;85:334–41.

17. Buechel FF Sr, Buechel FF Jr, Pappas MJ. Twenty-year evaluation of cementless mobile-bearing total ankle replacements. Clin Orthop Relat Res 2004; 424:19–26.

18. Haskell A, Mann RA. Perioperative complication rate of total ankle replacement is reduced by surgeon experience. Foot Ankle Int 2004;25:283–9.

19. Sturdee SW, Harris NJ, Farndon M. A prospective clinical and radiological review of 137 AES total ankle replacements over a 4-year period in a single centre. J Bone Joint Surg Br 2008;90(Suppl 3):495.

20. Álvarez-Goenaga F. Total ankle replacement: first 25 cases. Rev Esp Cir Ortop Traumatol 2008;52:224–32.

21. Lee KB, Cho SG, Hur CI, et al. Perioperative complications of Hintegra total ankle replacement: our initial 50 cases. Foot Ankle Int 2008;29:978–84.

22. Bai LB, Lee KB, Song EK, et al. Total ankle arthroplasty outcome comparison for post-traumatic and primary osteoarthritis. Foot Ankle Int 2010;31:1048–56.

23. Criswell BJ, Douglas K, Naik R, et al. High revision and reoperation rates using the Agility total ankle system. Clin Orthop Relat Res 2012;470:1980–6.

24. Pinar N, Vernet E, Bizot P, et al. Total ankle arthroplasty: total ankle arthroplasty in western France: influence of volume on complications and clinical outcome. Orthop Traumatol Surg Res 2012;98(Suppl):26–30.

25. Brunner S, Barg A, Knupp M, et al. The Scandinavian Total Ankle Replacement: long-term, eleven to fifteen-year, survivorship analysis of the prosthesis in seventy-two consecutive patients. J Bone Joint Surg Am 2013;95:711–8.

26. Lee KT, Lee YK, Young KW, et al. Perioperative complications and learning curve of the Mobility total ankle system. Foot Ankle Int 2013;34:210–4.

27. Schweitzer KM, Adams SB, Viens NA, et al. Early prospective clinical results of a modern fixed-bearing total ankle arthroplasty. J Bone Joint Surg Am 2013;95: 1002–11.

28. Glazebrook MA, Arsenault K, Dunbar M. Evidence-based classification of complications in total ankle arthroplasty. Foot Ankle Int 2009;30:945–9.

29. Gadd RJ, Barwick TW, Paling E, et al. Assessment of a three-grade classification of complications in total ankle replacement. Foot Ankle Int 2014;35:434–7.

30. Adams SB Jr, Demetracopoulos CA, Viens NA, et al. Comparison of extra-medullary versus intra-medullary referencing for tibial component alignment in total ankle arthroplasty. Foot Ankle Int 2013;34:1624–8.

31. Adams SB Jr, Spritzer CE, Hofstaetter SG, et al. Computer-assisted tibia preparation for total ankle arthroplasty: a cadaveric study. Int J Med Robot 2007;3: 336–40.

32. Sun SP, Su HW. Full-scale 3D preoperative planning system of the ankle joint replacement surgery with multimedia system. Smart Science 2014;2:80–4.

33. Hirao M, Oka K, Ikemoto S, et al. Use of a custom-made surgical guide in total ankle arthroplasty in rheumatoid arthritis cases. Tech Orthop 2014;29:102–11.

34. Berlet GC, Penner MJ, Lancianese S, et al. Total ankle arthroplasty accuracy and reproducibility using preoperative CT scan-derived, patient-specific guides. Foot Ankle Int 2014;35:665–76.

Total Ankle Replacement Survival Rates Based on Kaplan-Meier Survival Analysis of National Joint Registry Data

(●) CrossMark

Annette F.P. Bartel, DPM, MPH[a], Thomas S. Roukis, DPM, PhD[b],*

KEYWORDS

- Ankle evolutive system • Kaplan-Meier estimator • Prosthesis survival
- Scandinavian total ankle replacement • Total ankle arthroplasty

KEY POINTS

- National joint registries provide (1) timely feedback to surgeons and industry, (2) a sentinel for complications, (3) a reduction in patient morbidity, (4) the monitoring of new surgical techniques and implant technology, and (5) indications of poor implant design.

- The Kaplan-Meier estimator forecasts the probability of an event occurring over time with graphic representation of the resultant survival probability curve. The resultant survival curves based on the Kaplan-Meier estimator can be digitized and re-created to determine trends between registries.

- The survival rates of the 5152 primary total ankle replacements included over a 2- to 13-year period for all national joint registries were 0.94 (95% CI, 0.90–0.97) at 2 years, 0.87 (95% CI, 0.82–0.91) at 5 years, and 0.81 (95% CI, 0.74–0.88) at 10 years.

- National joint registries that included the Ankle Evolutive System (AES), Buechel-Pappas (BP), or Scandinavian Total Ankle Replacement (STAR) as greater than or equal to 35% of total prostheses implanted had survival rates between 0.78 and 0.89 at 5 years compared with registries with less than 35% of these implants, which were between 0.90 and 0.93 at 5 years.

- The STAR system should be implanted with caution until a dedicated revision system is developed and more robust long-term data are available supporting its continued use as a primary total ankle replacement (TAR).

Financial Disclosure: None reported.

Conflict of Interest: None reported.

[a] Gundersen Medical Foundation, 1900 South Avenue, La Crosse, WI 54601, USA; [b] Orthopaedic Center, Gundersen Health System, Mail Stop: CO2-006, 1900 South Avenue, La Crosse, WI 54601, USA

* Corresponding author.

E-mail address: tsroukis@gundersenhealth.org

Clin Podiatr Med Surg 32 (2015) 483–494

http://dx.doi.org/10.1016/j.cpm.2015.06.012

0891-8422/15/$ – see front matter © 2015 Elsevier Inc. All rights reserved.

podiatric.theclinics.com

INTRODUCTION

TAR has experienced clinical failure in early generations and accordingly was rendered nearly extinct. Dissatisfaction with ankle arthrodesis and the success of hip and knee arthroplasty, however, have renewed interest in TAR. Furthermore, the current growth of TAR can be credited to innovative surgeons and industry learning from the initial generations and modifying concepts to create a more biomechanically sound prostheses that can be inserted more reliably.[1]

The evolution of TAR is historically categorized into 3 generations based predominantly on (1) the number of components used, (2) the fixation method of the components to bone, and (3) the decades in use. Specifically, first-generation TARs (1960s through 1980s) consisted of a metallic component fixated to the tibia and polyethylene (PE) component fixated to the talus and vice versa that obtained bone fixation purely with polymethylmethacrylate (PMMA) cement. Limited dedicated instrumentation for prosthetic component implantation existed. Second-generation TARs (1980s through 2000s) consisted of 2 metallic or ceramic components, 1 affixed to the tibia and the other to the talus, secured to bone predominantly with PMMA cement, but some were fixated with metallic or biological porous coating. The PE insert was predominantly immobile and affixed to the undersurface of the tibial component, but some involved a partially mobile PE insert. Rudimentary instrumentation for prosthetic component implantation existed. Third-generation TARs (2000s to present day) consist of 2 metallic components, 1 affixed to the tibia and the other to the talus, secured to bone predominantly with metallic or biological porous coating and rarely PMMA cement. The PE insert predominantly involves a partially mobile design or, in a few designs, is immobile and affixed to the undersurface of the tibial component. Robust instrumentation for prosthetic component implantation exists, including intra- and extramedullary referencing, computer-assisted bone preparation, and CT scan–derived patient-specific guides.

It is generally believed that the first-generation TAR prostheses were far inferior to the second-generation prostheses, which in turn were inferior to the current third-generation prostheses.[1] Accordingly, TAR prosthesis longevity continues to be questioned and poorly understood, especially the effect, if any, the various design characteristics have had on prosthesis survival. It becomes more difficult to assess the effect of design characteristics because most TAR publications involve the prosthesis inventor, design team members, or paid company consultants. Therefore, strong potential for selection (inventor) and/or publication (conflict of interest) bias exists. For example, Labek and colleagues[2] studied the outcomes of second-generation TARs reported in clinical studies and national joint registries and identified significant selection (inventor) bias in approximately 50% of clinical studies. This effect was especially strong for the BP (Endotec, South Orange, New Jersey) and STAR (Waldemar Link, Hamburg, Germany/Small Bone Innovations, Morrisville, Pennsylvania/Stryker Orthopaedics, Mahwah, New Jersey) compared with national joint registry data. Additionally, a systematic review of primary implantation of the Agility Total Ankle Replacement System (DePuy Orthopaedics, Warsaw, Indiana) demonstrated that excluding the inventor increased the incidence of complications approximately 2-fold, from 6.6% (68/1033) to 12.2% (156/1279), implicating selection (inventor) bias.[3] Similarly, a systematic review of primary implantation of the STAR demonstrated that excluding the inventor or faculty consultants increased the incidence of complications more than 2-fold, from 5.6% (45/807) to 13.2% (224/1700), implicating selection (inventor) and publication (conflict of interest) bias.[4]

The implementation of national joint replacement registries worldwide would limit bias by providing large-scale prospective data collection and analysis of patient-related data and prosthetic component data and by including revision with explanation for failure as the primary outcome.[5] Currently, 33 national joint registries exist for all major orthopedic joints amenable to prosthetic implantation (http://www. arthroplastywatch.com/?page_id=5; last accessed August 23, 2014).

The Kaplan-Meier estimator is commonly used in orthopedic joint implant survival analysis in peer-reviewed articles and in worldwide joint registries.[6,7] The Kaplan-Meier estimator forecasts the probability of an event occurring over time, with graphic representation of the resultant survival probability curve. The survival probability of each time interval is calculated as a product of the conditional properties of surviving time until a chosen time. The survival times are censored when a patient is lost to follow-up, experiences death, or does not experience the event, such as a revision. Dobbs[8] first used this estimate for implant revision in 1980, reporting on 400 Stanmore total hip arthroplasties (Centre for Biomedical Engineering, Royal National Orthopaedic Hospital, Middlesex, England). Although the Kaplan-Meier estimator has become a more common reporting statistic in orthopedic literature, it is not consistently reported for direct comparison of implant survival and trends at any point in time, such as 1 year, 5 years, or 10 years.

To date, no study has been performed that specifically compares TAR prosthesis survival between national joint registries. Therefore, this article re-creates primary TAR survival curves among published national joint registry data sets using the Kaplan-Meier estimator to determine the survival rates between registries at 1-year intervals. The number and type of TAR prosthesis implanted also were recorded and reported.

METHODS

The 33 listed joint registries identified worldwide were searched in detail (http://www. arthroplastywatch.com/?page_id=5; last accessed August 23, 2014). Additionally, 2 general Internet-based search engines, Google and Google Scholar, were used to search for additional national joint registry publications involving TAR based on a prior publication of this topic.[5]

TAR survival was defined as retention of the prosthesis without revision, removal, or exchange of part of or the entire prosthesis. The national joint registries' specific definitions of revision were noted and are described in **Table 1** for consistency, although slight variations were apparent between registries.

Next, each national joint registry was evaluated for the presence of a Kaplan-Meier TAR survival curve and values reported. The Kaplan-Meier data points were extracted from the included articles as a portable document format (PDF) and imported into the software Digitizelt (http://www.digitizeit.de/; last accessed August 23, 2014) (Digitizelt, Braunschweig, Germany) for hand digitization.[9] Censored events were excluded from digitization due to poor resolution quality to differentiate the number of events. The digitized coordinates of time (X axis) and survival probability (Y axis) were exported into Microsoft Excel 2010 (Microsoft, Redmond, Washington) for further analysis. Time increments of 1 year each were defined and extracted from each data set to re-create the Kaplan-Meier curve. If a Kaplan-Meier curve was not provided, the reported values were recorded according to 1-year increments.

RESULTS

Australia[10]; England, Wales, and Northern Ireland[11]; Finland[12]; New Zealand[13–15]; Norway[16,17]; and Sweden[18–20] had data available from their national joint registry data sets that involved TAR and had enough information to generate Kaplan-Meier

Table 1	
Definitions of failure of a total ankle replacement as reported in national joint registries	
National Joint Registry	Definition of Total Ankle Replacement Failure
New Zealand Joint Registry[13–15]	New operation in previously operated ankle joint with 1 or more components exchanged, added, removed or manipulated
Norwegian Arthroplasty Register[16,17]	Removal or exchange of a part of implant or the whole implant
Swedish Ankle Registry[18–20]	Exchange or extraction of 1 or more of the 3 prosthetic components with the exception of incidental exchange of the PE insert
AOA National Joint Replacement Registry[10]	Revision procedures are reoperations of previous ankle replacements where 1 or more of the prosthetic components are replaced or removed or another component is added. Revisions include reoperations of primary partial, primary total, or previous revision procedures.
National Joint Registry for England, Wales and Northern Ireland[11]	None provided
Finnish Arthroplasty Register[12]	One component or the whole implant removed or exchanged

survival curves. Among the included registries, 5152 primary and 591 TAR revisions were reported over a 2- to 13-year period. Primary TAR survival rates from all national joint registries were 0.94 (95% CI, 0.90–0.97) at 2 years, 0.87 (95% CI, 0.82–0.91) at 5 years, and 0.81 (95% CI, 0.74–0.88) at 10 years.

The authors determined that Kaplan-Meier estimator curves could be reliably reproduced to plot survival trends for evaluation and determine the Kaplan-Meier estimator at any point of time (**Fig. 1**). The Finnish Arthroplasty Register[12] had no difference between re-created value of 0.83 and 0.83 (95% CI, 0.81–0.86) reported at 5 years. The New Zealand Joint Registry[13–15] had no discrepancy of values between stated and re-created plots (0.99 at 1 year, 0.93 at 5 years, and 0.90 at 7 years, with reported values censoring deceased patients at time of death). The Norwegian Arthroplasty Register[16,17] had no difference in stated and re-created values at 5 years of 0.89 (stated 95% CI, 0.84–0.93). The Swedish Ankle Registry[18–20] demonstrated minor differences between stated and re-created plots of 0.92 re-created and 0.94 (95% CI, 0.93–0.95) reported at 1 year, 0.78 re-created and 0.81 (95% CI, 0.79–0.83) reported at 5 years, and 0.66 re-created and 0.69 (95% CI, 0.67–0.71) reported at 10 years. The Australian Orthopaedic Association (AOA) National Joint Replacement Registry[10] and National Joint Registry for England, Wales and Northern Ireland[11] provided reported data without supporting survival curves and accordingly these could not be evaluated.

The New Zealand Joint Registry[13–15] reports a 13-year analysis on 944 primary TARs performed (**Table 2**); 53 revisions and 6 re-revisions were performed out of the primary TAR group. The most common prosthesis implanted was the Mobility Total Ankle System (DePuy, Leeds, England) (n = 443, 47%) followed by the Salto Mobile version ankle prosthesis (Tornier, Saint-Martin, France) (n = 316, 33%). The calculated Kaplan-Meier estimator was 0.98 at 2 years, 0.93 at 5 years, and 0.86 at 10 years.

The Norwegian Arthroplasty Register[16,17] reports a 13-year analysis on 720 primary TARs performed (see **Table 2**); 216 revisions were reported. The most common

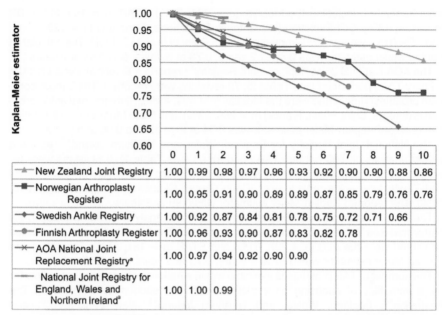

Fig. 1. Survival of TARs based on registry data of re-created Kaplan-Meier estimators. [a]Kaplan-Meier estimators as reported without a survival curve re-created. (*Data from* New Zealand Joint Registry,[13–15] Norwegian Arthroplasty Register,[16,17] Swedish Ankle Registry,[18–20] Finnish Arthroplasty Register,[12] AOA National Joint Replacement Registry,[10] and National Joint Registry for England, Wales and Northern Ireland.[11])

prosthesis implanted was the STAR (n = 537, 75%). The calculated Kaplan-Meier estimator was 0.91 at 2 years, 0.89, at 5 years, and 0.76 at 10 years.

The Swedish Ankle Registry[18–20] reports a 12-year analysis on 871 primary TARs performed (see **Table 2**); 208 revisions were reported. A wide variety of prosthesis

Table 2
National joint registries evaluated, including total ankle replacement prostheses studies, implantation start, final study year, and reported revisions

Registry	Publication Year	Study Start Year	Study Final Year	Total Ankle Replacements (n)	Revisions Reported
New Zealand Joint Registry[13–15]	2013	2000	2012	944	59
Norwegian Arthroplasty Register[16,17]	2013	2000	2012	720	216
Swedish Ankle Registry[18–20]	2013	2000	2012	871	208
AOA National Joint Replacement Registry[10]	2013	2007	2012	1127	72
National Joint Registry for England, Wales and Northern Ireland[11]	2012	2010	2012	999	9
Finnish Arthroplasty Register[12]	2010	2000	2010	491	27
Total	—	—	—	5152	591

were implanted, including the Mobility (n = 234, 27%), STAR (n = 194, 22%), BP (n = 154, 18%), CCI Evolution (Implantcast, Buxtehude, Germany) (n = 128, 15%), and AES (Transysteme-JMT Implants, Nimes, France) (n = 117, 13%). The calculated Kaplan-Meier estimator was 0.87 at 2 years, 0.78 at 5 years, and 0.66 at 9 years.

The AOA National Joint Replacement Registry[10] reports a 6-year analysis on 1127 primary TARs performed (see **Table 2**); 72 revisions were reported. The 2 most common prosthesis implanted were the Mobility (n = 494, 44%), Hintegra total ankle prosthesis (Integra, Saint Priest, France) (n = 256, 23%), and Salto Mobile (n = 198, 18%). The reported Kaplan-Meier estimator was 0.94 at 2 years and 0.90 at 5 years.

The National Joint Registry for England, Wales and Northern Ireland[11] reports a 5-year analysis on 999 primary TARs performed (see **Table 2**); 9 revisions were reported. The 2 most common prosthesis implanted were the Mobility (n = 539, 54%) and Zenith total ankle replacement (Corin Group, Cirencester, England) (n = 210, 21%). The reported Kaplan-Meier estimator was 0.99 at 2 years.

The Finnish Arthroplasty Register[12] reports a 7-year analysis on 491 primary TARs performed (see **Table 2**); 27 revisions were reported. The 2 most common prostheses implanted were the AES (n = 298, 61%) and STAR (n = 181, 37%). The calculated Kaplan-Meier estimator was 0.87 at 2 years, 0.78 at 5 years, and 0.66 at 9 years.

The number of TAR prostheses available within a national joint registry may allow for more versatility of choosing an implant specific for each patient (**Table 3**). The Australian[10]; England, Wales, and Northern Ireland[11]; New Zealand[13–15]; and Norwegian[16,17] registries included greater than or equal to 7 TAR designs and the cumulative Kaplan-Meier estimator ranged from 0.89 to 0.93 when 5-year survival data were provided. When the AES and STAR were greater than or equal to 35% of the TAR prosthesis included within the registry,[12,16–20] the Kaplan-Meier was 0.78 to 0.89 at 5 years, whereas for registries with less than 35% of these prostheses included, the Kaplan-Meier was 0.90 to 0.93 at 5 years.[10,11,13–15]

DISCUSSION

The purpose of this study was to re-create primary TAR survival curves among available national joint registry data sets using the Kaplan-Meier estimator to determine the survival rates between registries at 1-year intervals. A total of 6 national joint registry data sets were identified that included TAR prostheses.

A review of the data allow for some generalized observations. First, the definitions of TAR failure as stated in the included registries were similar and consisted of removal or exchange of a part of or the whole prosthesis, excluding incidental exchange of the PE insert (see **Table 1**). The National Joint Registry of England, Wales and Northern Ireland[11] did not provide a definition of revision within their registry data. These definitions should continue to be monitored for consistency when included in future implants survival analysis to predictably exclude secondary procedures or PE insert exchanges as revisions.[21]

Second, the included studies spanned 2 to 13 years of national joint registry data evaluating 5152 primary and 591 TAR revisions recorded, demonstrating a lengthy follow-up period with robust patient population for evaluation. A lengthy follow-up and patient population demonstrate the generational trends apparent within the evolving TAR industry and surgeon learning curve during both primary and revision TAR.[1] For example, a systematic review of TAR prosthesis use in national joint registries was able to identify 3 general patterns of prosthesis use over a 10-year period: (1) minimal use, (2) initial embracement followed by abrupt disuse, and (3) embracement with sustained growth. Further analysis of national joint registries for those TAR prostheses

Table 3
Number of total ankle replacements implanted per prosthesis type and national joint registry

Total Ankle Replacement System/Prosthesis Type	AES[a]	Agility[b]	BOX[c]	BP[d]	CCI[e]	ESKA[f]	Hintegra[g]	Inbone II[h]	Mobility[i]	Ramses[j]	Rebalance[k]	Salto Mobile[l]	STAR[m]	Taric[n]	Zenith[o]	Total
New Zealand Joint Registry[13–15]	—	119	4	—	—	—	5	—	443	11	—	316	46	—	—	944
Norwegian Arthroplasty Register[16,17]	3	—	—	58	—	11	—	85	—	—	15	11	537	—	—	720
Swedish Ankle Registry[18–20]	117	—	—	154	128	—	—	234	—	—	44	—	194	—	—	871
AOA National Joint Replacement Registry[10]	—	2	93	59	4	1	256	—	494	—	—	198	13	—	7	1127
National Joint Registry for England, Wales and Northern Ireland[11]	—	—	72	—	—	—	43	2	539	—	15	63	54	1	210	999
Finnish Arthroplasty Register[12]	298	—	—	—	—	—	12	—	—	—	—	—	181	—	—	491

[a] AES (Transysteme-JMT Implants, Nimes, France).
[b] Agility (DePuy Orthopaedics, Inc, Warsaw, IN).
[c] Bologna-Oxford (Finsbury, Leatherhead, United Kingdom).
[d] BP (Endotec, South Orange, NJ).
[e] CCI Evolution (Implantcast GMBH Lüneburger Schanze Buxtehude, Germany).
[f] ESKA (GmbH & Co, Lübeck, Germany).
[g] Hintegra (Integra, Saint Priest, France).
[h] Inbone II (Wright Medical Technology, Memphis, TN).
[i] Mobility (DePuy UK, Leeds, England).
[j] Ramses (Laboratoire Fournitures Hospitalières Industrie, Heimsbrunn, France).
[k] Rebalance (Biomet UK Ltd, Bridgend, South Wales, England).
[l] Salto Mobile Version (Tornier, Saint-Martin, France).
[m] STAR (Waldemar Link, Hamburg, Germany/Small Bone Innovations, Inc, Morrisville, PA/Stryker Orthopaedics, Mahwah, NJ).
[n] Taric (Implantcast GmbH, Buxtehude, Germany).
[o] Zenith (Corin Group PLC, Cirencester, England).

that were initially embraced only to abruptly fall into disuse may help warn surgeons, industry, and the public about prosthesis design flaws or specific surgeon concerns that led to the abrupt disuse. A prime example of the initial embracement followed by abrupt disuse trend is the withdrawal of the AES prosthesis after identification of a higher than expected complication rate. Ultimately it was determined that the use of hydroxyapatite coating was the major cause of the severe aseptic osteolysis seen with the AES prosthesis (http://webarchive.nationalarchives.gov.uk/20141205150130/http://www.mhra.gov.uk/home/groups/dts-bs/documents/medicaldevicealert/con174792. pdf; last accessed August 23, 2014), and industries producing TAR systems with this coating should take heed to avoiding repeating the past. Furthermore, current TAR prostheses that are in a sustained growth period should be carefully evaluated to identify any trends in use that may be a cause for concern prior to widespread abrupt disuse. For example, analysis of the Salto Mobile prosthesis across national joint registries up to 2011 indicates it is has been embraced and is undergoing sustained growth.[5] The Salto Mobile prosthesis first appeared in the Norwegian Arthroplasty Register[16] in 2012, however, and was abruptly replaced by the fixed-bearing Salto Talaris and Salto Talaris XT total ankle prostheses (Tornier, Bloomington, Minnesota) in 2013.[22] The rationale for this abrupt conversion from the mobile to PE fixed-bearing version of the same TAR system, especially when the other TAR systems included in the registry have relatively consistent use over a much longer time period, is intriguing but unknown. Analysis over time within this and other registries may clarify the reason for this trend and herald the importance of scrutiny of primary TAR implantation trends in national joint registries.

Third, for national joint registries that included the AES, BP, or STAR as greater than or equal to 35% of total primary TARs implanted, the survival rate was 0.78 to 0.89 at 5 years compared with registries with less than 35% of these prostheses, where the survival rate was 0.90 to 0.93 at 5 years (**Fig. 2**). The BP was withdrawn from use in 2009 and the AES in 2010 for the reasons discussed previously.[5] The version of the STAR available for use in the United States is a single-coated titanium plasma spray on the metallic components.[4] This is an important consideration because the Norwegian Arthroplasty Register demonstrated a difference in survival between the hydroxyapatite single-coated and partially titanium–calcium phosphate double-coated version compared with the double-coated design that demonstrated better results specific to incidence of prosthetic loosening.[16,17] This same study found no difference in revision incidence between both versions of the uncemented STAR and the cemented Thompson Parkridge Richards ankle prosthesis, which was a first-generation prosthesis removed from use in 1997.[16,17] Furthermore, the Finnish Arthroplasty Register[12] demonstrated a parallel and steep incidence of revision between the double-coated version of the STAR and the AES, which, as noted, has been withdrawn from use due to higher than expected frequency of osteolytic lesions and component failure.[23] Finally, the second generation of the STAR has been demonstrated to have a similar survival rate as the first-generation version of the STAR that involved an all-PE tibial component secured with PMMA cement and a stainless steel metallic talar component[24] irrespective of age at time of implantation[25] or etiology.[26,27] This is concerning because there has been apparent widespread adoption of the porous titanium single-coated STAR in the United States (http://www.businesswire.com/news/home/20120411006339/en/Independent-Survey-U.S.-Foot-Ankle-Surgeons-Affirms; last accessed August 23, 2014). Unfortunately, multiple studies have demonstrated that the complication rate and incidence of revision are even higher than previously reported for the STAR prosthesis. Brunner and colleagues[28] presented 10.8- to 14.9-year results for 77 primary STAR prosthesis with a single coating of hydroxyapatite;

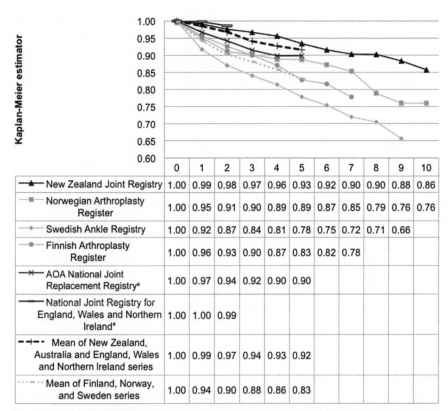

Fig. 2. Survival of TARs based on registry data of re-created Kaplan-Meier estimators separating registries that included greater than or equal to 35% of total implants as AES and/or STAR prostheses (*black lines*) and registries that included less than 35% of total implants as AES and/or STAR prostheses (*gray lines*). [a]Kaplan-Meier estimators as reported without a survival curve re-created. (*Data from* New Zealand Joint Registry,[13–15] Norwegian Arthroplasty Register,[16,17] Swedish Ankle Registry,[18–20] Finnish Arthroplasty Register,[12] AOA National Joint Replacement Registry,[10] and National Joint Registry for England, Wales and Northern Ireland.[11])

29 (38%) of the 77 prostheses had a revision and the survival rates were 0.71 at 10 years and 0.46 at 14 years. Similarly, Clough and colleagues[29] presented 13- to 19-year results of 200 consecutive primary STAR prostheses and reported a survival rate of 0.77 (95% CI, 66.4–87.3) at 15 years. Furthermore, the complete abandonment of the STAR prosthesis in the New Zealand Joint Registry[13–15] and near-complete disuse evident in the Finnish Arthroplasty Register[12] should be carefully considered. These findings support the critical evaluation of prosthesis implantation and revision trends through national joint registries with expansion to include modes of failure as an understanding of the actual incidence of revision, the most common etiology leading to failure, and the revision options for each prosthesis system is critical to optimizing patient outcome.

Fourth, survival curves of re-created Kaplan-Meier estimators can be reliably reconstructed as demonstrated (see **Fig. 1**) and matched to the reported estimators. All values re-created are exact, as demonstrated by Finish,[12] New Zealand,[13–15] and Norwegian[16,17] registries or within the stated 95% CI, as demonstrated by the Swedish[18–20] registry data. When the survival curve is included in the registry data and re-created in a reproducible standard method,[9] further data points can be inferred to compare time intervals that may not be clearly stated. The number and reasons of specific implant failure are lacking, which allows for re-creation of the TAR prosthesis survival curves and the ability to infer trends, such as minimal use, disuse, or sustained use, that may be related to failure rates per implant design and collectively per generation.[5,30,31]

LIMITATIONS

Kaplan-Meier survival curves are commonly used in orthopedic literature for implant survival data but are not without limitation. The Kaplan-Meier estimator is designed to estimate the probability of an event to eventually occur for all patients, such as death. This assumption does not hold true for those with a prosthetic joint replacement where component loosening or failure may occur before death. The estimator has the ability to overestimate probability of an event occurring with time in the presence of competing risks, such as revision, long-term component loosening, or failure in general as an endpoint[6,7]

The authors recommend that future peer-reviewed studies and national joint registry data include a Kaplan-Meier survival curve with the numbers at risk for complete parallel of survival outcomes. Revision rates by specific TAR prosthesis were not always reported, leading to uncertainty of prosthesis longevity based on individual design, PE insert characteristics, or other features. Future inclusion of revision rates specific to prosthesis type would lead to further understanding of TAR survival or failure trends, thereby benefiting patients, surgeons, and industry because changes could be made to the specific TAR that may ultimately improve prosthesis survival.

Reconstruction of Kaplan-Meier curves can provide further information about TAR survival but not without limitations.[8] First, a Kaplan-Meier curve does not separate information about various subgroups but, instead, pools data together over differing covariants that may affect survival, leading to aggregation bias. Second, reliability of the reconstructed data relies on the quality of initial input of information and the level of information provided by the publication. Low-quality PDF images can lead to difficulty extracting accurate data via digitization and were the result of not digitizing censored events. Future publications and national joint registry data should strive to include time-to-event outcomes, Kaplan-Meier curves with numbers at risk, and total number of events to be transparent in data re-creation or worldwide trends.

Limited peer-reviewed publications are available for prosthesis survival analysis and are often accompanied with significant selection (inventor) bias and must be interpreted with caution. The use of national joint registry data is not without error but is reported prospectively for the participating countries in a similar process involved with the peer-review process leading to publication.

SUMMARY

National joint registry data collectively provide unique information about primary TAR and subsequent revision to collectively analyze prosthesis survival. When provided, survival curves based on the Kaplan-Meier estimator can be digitized and re-created with accuracy. Overall, 5152 primary and 591 TAR revisions were included over a 2- to 13-year period, with prosthesis survival rates for all national joint registries of 0.94 (95% CI, 0.90–0.97) at 2 years, 0.87 (95% CI, 0.82–0.91) at 5 years, and 0.81 (95% CI, 0.74–0.88) at 10 years. For national joint registries that included the AES, BP, and/or STAR as greater than or equal to 35% of total prostheses implanted, the survival rate was 0.78 to 0.89 at 5 years compared with registries with less than 35% of these prostheses at 0.90 to 0.93 at 5 years. Both the AES and BP have been withdrawn from the market and, based on available national registry data, the STAR has fallen into worldwide disuse. This finding supports the critical evaluation of primary TAR implantation and revision trends through national joint registries with expansion to include modes of prosthesis failure. The STAR system should be implanted with caution until a dedicated revision system is developed and more robust long-term data are available supporting its continued use as a primary TAR. Future studies and national joint registry data sets should continue to strive for completion of data presentation to include revision definitions, modes of failure, time of failure, and patients lost to follow-up or death for complete accuracy of the Kaplan-Meier estimator.

REFERENCES

1. Gougoulias N, Maffulli N. History of total ankle replacement. Clin Podiatr Med Surg 2013;30:1–20.
2. Labek G, Thaler M, Janda W, et al. Revision rates after total joint replacement: cumulative results from worldwide joint register datasets. J Bone Joint Surg Br 2011; 93:293–7.
3. Roukis TS. Incidence of revision after primary implantation of the agility total ankle replacement system: a systematic review. J Foot Ankle Surg 2012;51: 198–204.
4. Prissel MA, Roukis TS. Incidence of revision after primary implantation of the Scandinavian total ankle replacement system: a systematic review. Clin Podiatr Med Surg 2013;30:237–50.
5. Roukis TS, Prissel MA. Registry data trends of total ankle replacement use. J Foot Ankle Surg 2013;52:728–35.
6. Biau DJ, Latouche A, Porcher R. Competing events influence estimated survival probability: when is Kaplan-Meier analysis appropriate? Clin Orthop Relat Res 2007;462:229–33.
7. Biau DJ, Hamadouche M. Estimating implant survival in the presence of competing risks. Int Orthop 2011;35:151–5.
8. Dobbs HS. Survivorship of total hip replacements. J Bone Joint Surg Br 1980;62: 168–73.
9. Guyot P, Ades AE, Ouwens MJ, et al. Enhanced secondary analysis of survival data: reconstructing the data from published Kaplan-Meier survival curves. BMC Med Res Methodol 2012;12:9. Available at: http://www.biomedcentral.com/1471-2288/12/9. Accessed July 27, 2014.
10. Australian Orthopaedic Association. National Joint Replacement Registry, Demographics and Outcome of Ankle Arthroplasty Supplementary Report 2013. Available at: https://aoanjrr.dmac.adelaide.edu.au/en/annual-reports-2013. Accessed August 23, 2014.
11. National Joint Registry for England, Wales and Northern Ireland, 9th Annual report of prothesis used in hip, knee, and ankle replacement procedures 2012. Available at: http://www.njrcentre.org.uk/njrcentre/Reports,Publicationsand Minutes/Annualreports/tabid/86/Default.aspx. Accessed August 23, 2014.
12. Skyttä ET, Koivu H, Eskelinen A, et al. Total ankle replacement: a population-based study of 515 cases from the Finnish Arthroplasty Register. Acta Orthop 2010;81:114–8.
13. Hosman AH, Mason RB, Hobbs T, et al. A New Zealand National Joint Registry review of 202 total ankle replacements followed for up to 6 years. Acta Orthop 2007;78:584–91.

14. The New Zealand Joint Registry Annual Report 2013. Available at: www.nzoa.org. nz/system/files/NJR%2014%20Year%20Report.pdf. Accessed August 23, 2014.
15. Tomlinson M, Harrison M. The New Zealand Joint Registry: report of 11-year data for ankle arthroplasty. Foot Ankle Clin 2012;17:719–23.
16. Norwegian Arthroplasty Register 2013. Available at: http://nrlweb.ihelse.net/ Rapporter/Rapport2013.pdf. Accessed August 23, 2014.
17. Fevang BTS, Lie SA, Havelin LI, et al. 257 ankle arthroplasties performed in Norway between 1994 and 2005. Acta Orthop 2007;78:575–83.
18. The Swedish Ankle Register for total ankle replacements and ankle arthrodeses: Annual report for 2012. Available at: www.swedankle.se/pdf/rapporter/annual-report-2012.pdf. Accessed August 23, 2014.
19. Henricson A, Nilsson JÅ, Carlsson A. 10-year survival of total ankle arthroplasties: a report on 780 cases from the Swedish Ankle Register. Acta Orthop 2011;82: 655–9.
20. Henricson A, Skoog A, Carlsson Å. The Swedish Ankle Arthroplasty Register: an analysis of 531 arthroplasties between 1993 and 2005. Acta Orthop 2007;78: 569–74.
21. Henricson A, Carlsson Å, Rydholm U. What is a revision of total ankle replacement? Foot Ankle Surg 2011;17:99–102.
22. Norwegian Arthroplasty Register 2014. Available at: http://nrlweb.ihelse.net/ Rapporter/Rapport2014.pdf. Accessed August 23, 2014.
23. Dalat F, Barnoud R, Fessy MH, et al. Histologic study of periprosthetic osteolytic lesions after AES total ankle replacement. A 22 case series. Orthop Traumatol Surg Res 2013;99:S285–95.
24. Kofoed H. Scandinavian total ankle replacement (STAR). Clin Orthop Relat Res 2004;(424):73–9.
25. Kofoed H, Lundberg-Jensen A. Ankle arthroplasty in patients younger and older than 50 years. A prospective series with long-term follow-up. Foot Ankle Int 1999; 20:501–6.
26. Kofoed H. Cylindrical cemented ankle arthroplasty: a prospective series with long-term follow-up. Foot Ankle Int 1995;16:474–9.
27. Kofoed H, Sørensen TS. Ankle arthroplasty for rheumatoid arthritis and osteoarthritis. Prospective long-term study of cemented replacements. J Bone Joint Surg Br 1998;80:328–32.
28. Brunner S, Barg A, Knupp M. The Scandinavian total ankle replacement: long-term, eleven to fifteen-year, survivorship analysis of the prosthesis in seventy-two consecutive patients. J Bone Joint Surg Am 2013;95:711–8.
29. Clough T, Talbot C, Siney P, et al. 13–19 year results of a consecutive series of 200 Scandinavian Total Ankle Replacements (STAR): the Wrightington Experience. Bone Joint J 2014;96(Suppl 2):32.
30. Pappas MJ, Buechel FF Sr. Failure modes of current total ankle replacement systems. Clin Podiatr Med Surg 2013;30:123–43.
31. Sadoghi P, Roush G, Kastner N, et al. Failure modes for total ankle arthroplasty: a statistical analysis of the Norwegian Arthroplasty Register. Arch Orthop Trauma Surg 2014;134(10):1361–8.

Arthroscopic Management of Complications Following Total Ankle Replacement

Tun Hing Lui, MBBS (HK), FRCS (Edin), FHKAM, FHKCOS[a,*],
Thomas S. Roukis, DPM, PhD[b]

KEYWORDS

- Agility total ankle replacement system • HINTEGRA ankle prosthesis • Revision
- Salto Talaris total ankle replacement system
- Scandinavian total ankle replacement system • Total ankle arthroplasty

KEY POINTS

- With the advance in foot and ankle arthroscopy and endoscopy, the list of pathologic conditions that can be dealt with through these approaches is expanding. There is great potential for managing the complications of total ankle replacement arthroscopically and/or endoscopically, and these procedures can be summarized into 3 groups.
- Group 1 includes procedures of the ankle joint proper with close proximity to the articular components of the total ankle replacement. This group includes arthroscopic medial, lateral, anterior, and posterior gutter soft tissue and osseous debridement.
- Group 2 includes procedures of the tibia and talus with close proximity to the nonarticular parts of the total ankle replacement. This group includes endoscopic cyst curettage and impaction bone grafting of the immediate periprosthetic osteolysis and cyst formations.
- Group 3 includes procedures that are away from the total ankle replacement. This group includes posterior tibial tendon endoscopic decompression, endoscopic curettage and grafting of the fibular bone cyst, endoscopic gastrocnemius release, midtarsal and subtalar arthroscopic debridement, arthroscopic subtalar or triple arthrodesis, and endoscopic lateral calcaneal decompression.
- Foot and ankle arthroscopic and endoscopic procedures have many potential applications to manage complications after total ankle replacement. However, these remain master arthroscopist procedures and should be performed by foot and ankle surgeons who perform them with regularity until further large-scale studies are available to guide these therapies.

[a] Department of Orthopaedics and Traumatology, North District Hospital, 9 Po Kin Road, Sheung Shui, New Territories, Hong Kong SAR, China; [b] Orthopaedic Center, Gundersen Health System, Mail Stop: CO2-006, 1900 South Avenue, La Crosse, WI 54601, USA
* Corresponding author.
E-mail address: luithderek@yahoo.co.uk

Clin Podiatr Med Surg 32 (2015) 495–508
http://dx.doi.org/10.1016/j.cpm.2015.06.016   **podiatric.theclinics.com**
0891-8422/15/$ – see front matter © 2015 Elsevier Inc. All rights reserved.

INTRODUCTION

Total ankle replacement (TAR) has become more popular and is hoped to solve the long-term problems associated with ankle arthrodesis, specifically accelerated degeneration of adjacent joints that are difficult to treat; alterations in gait mechanics even with a well-aligned ankle arthrodesis; limitations in activity, especially ones requiring exposure to uneven ground and stairs/inclines; and painful nonunion of the arthrodesis site. Modern TAR systems consist of 3 components: a metallic baseplate affixed to the tibia, a domed- or condylar-shaped metallic component that resurfaces the talus, and a fixed-bearing or mobile-bearing surface made of ultrahigh molecular weight polyethylene (UHMWPE) interposed between the tibial and talar components. Although the ideal balance between constraint and stability remains unknown, the results of contemporary total ankle systems using semiconstrained components with biological ongrowth for fixation suggest a significant advance in prosthetic design over the previous generations.[1]

Despite the advance in the design of the TAR systems, high complication rates of greater than 50% have been seen at intermediate- and long-term follow-up evaluations, and mean revision rates of 21% for TAR at the time of a 5-year follow-up have been reported.[2] There is an endless list of possible complications associated with TAR, including aseptic loosening, especially of the talar component; osteolysis and osteonecrosis of the talus; arthrofibrosis; soft tissue and osseous impingement; instability; intraoperative or postoperative periprosthetic fracture; implant failure; subsidence especially of the talus component; deep periprosthetic infection and wound healing problems; development of ossifications/osteophytes, especially in the area of the medial malleolus or the anterior part of the ankle, leading to impingement and loss of mobility; and tendo-Achilles contracture leading to equinus.[3,4]

Glazebrook and colleagues[5] summarized the complications into 9 groups:

1. Intraoperative fracture
2. Postoperative fracture
3. Wound-healing problems
4. Deep periprosthetic infection
5. Aseptic loosening
6. Nonunion
7. Implant failure
8. Subsidence
9. Technical error

They are classified into 3 grades of severity. High-grade complications of implant failure, aseptic loosening, and deep infection were associated with high failure rates for TAR. Medium-grade complications of technical error, subsidence, and postoperative fracture were associated with moderate failure rates. Low-grade complications of intraoperative fracture and problems with wound healing demonstrated negligible failure rates.[5,6] However, some investigators thought that most complications associated with TAR have a significant impact on the life span of a TAR; Glazebrook and colleagues's[5] proposed 3-tier system did not reliably reflect the impact of the complications.[7,8]

OVERVIEW OF POTENTIAL APPLICATIONS OF ARTHROSCOPY AND ENDOSCOPY IN MANAGEMENT OF COMPLICATIONS FOLLOWING TOTAL ANKLE REPLACEMENT

With the advance in foot and ankle arthroscopy and endoscopy, the list of pathologic conditions that can be dealt with using these approaches is expanding. There is great potential to manage the complications of TAR arthroscopically. The arthroscopic procedures can be summarized into 3 groups:

1. Procedures of the ankle joint proper with close proximity to the articular components of the TAR
2. Procedures of the tibia and talus with close proximity to the nonarticular parts of the TAR
3. Procedures that are away from the TAR

The arthroscopic and open procedures can be comprehensive and not mutually exclusive. In cases with incorrectly addressed hindfoot misalignment and/or incorrectly positioned prosthesis components, pain may remain postoperatively because of biomechanical imbalance and asymmetrical load. The pain is mostly localized on the medial side, the so-called *medial pain syndrome*. It has been classified into type I medial impingement/contracture of medial ligaments, type II valgus deformity, type III varus deformity, and type IV combined varus-valgus deformity.[9] Arthroscopic debridement of the medial ankle gutter can be coupled with calcaneal realignment osteotomy. Moreover, lateral ankle impingement pain associated with valgus heel after TAR can be managed by posterior calcaneal osteotomy and endoscopic lateral calcaneal decompression.[10,11] The contraindications include those conditions that need removal or exchange of the TAR such as for aseptic loosening of the prosthesis or deep periprosthetic infection.

PROCEDURES OF THE ANKLE JOINT PROPER WITH CLOSE PROXIMITY TO THE ARTICULAR COMPONENTS OF THE TOTAL ANKLE REPLACEMENT

This group of arthroscopic procedures mainly includes gutter procedures and deals with pathologic conditions of the anterior, posterior, medial, and lateral gutters of the ankle. In contrast to the usual ankle arthroscopy, there is TAR in situ. Surgeons should pay particular attention to avoid damage to the prosthesis, especially the polyethylene liner during the procedure; instrumentation between the articular surfaces should be avoided.[12,13] With careful placement of the portal incisions and care with placement of the arthroscopic devices, iatrogenic damage can be avoided.[12] Standard anterior ankle arthroscopy with the anterior-medial and anterior-lateral portals is usually sufficient to deal with pathologic conditions of the anterior, medial, and lateral gutters. Posterior ankle endoscopy[14] or posterior ankle arthroscopy[15,16] can be used to address myriad pathologic conditions of the posterior gutter.

Medial Gutter

Medial impingement is a frequent complication following TAR. It can be soft tissue or osseous impingement or both. It can be a result of prosthesis design, technical error of medially placed tibial prosthesis, oversizing of the prosthesis, loosening of the prosthesis, inadequate/no prophylactic gutter resection, failure to address hindfoot mal-alignment and heterotopic bone formation.[12,17,18] Moreover, impingement pain can occur in cases of residual ankle instability where in the prosthesis glides into the malleolus leading to friction and wear.[13] Preexisting medial joint arthritis, model of TAR, or an intraoperative fracture of the medial malleolus do not influence the incidence of medial impingement.[17–19] The use of prosthesis designs like the Agility Total Ankle Replacement System (DePuy Synthes Orthopedics, Inc, Warsaw, IN, USA) that replace medial and lateral recesses may not prevent impingement symptoms as the impingement can occur as a result of heterotopic bone formation.[19] Moreover, soft tissue impingement can still occur even if the medial and lateral recesses are replaced.

Rippstein and colleagues[20] reported medial ankle pain as a complication of both the Scandinavian Total Ankle Replacement System (Stryker Orthopedics, Inc, Mahwah, NJ, USA) and the Buechel-Pappas (Endotec, South Orange, NJ, USA). This complication may be caused by the cylindrical shape of the talar component. This idea has not been proven yet but has been addressed in newer designs, such as the Salto Mobile Version prosthesis (Tornier NV, Amsterdam, The Netherlands) and the HINTEGRA Ankle Prosthesis (Newdeal, Lyon, France/Integra, Plainsboro, NJ, USA).[19] Kim and colleagues[21] reported an increased incidence of medial soft tissue impingement in those patients with a medial ligament releasing procedure during TAR. This effect should be studied further.

Besides the intra-articular impingement, there are possibilities of extra-articular posteromedial and anteromedial pain syndromes. The posteromedial pain syndrome is caused by impingement of the posterior tibial tendon and is discussed in the following section. The chronic anteromedial pain is located in the anterior-medial soft tissues, outside of the ankle joint itself, and can radiate proximally into the medial malleolus. This pain is probably related to increased medial soft tissue tension. Surgical release of the deltoid ligament is indicated when repeated local injection is not successful. During anterior ankle arthroscopy, the deep deltoid fibers can be transacted with the anteromedial portal as the instrumentation portal. Caution should be paid to preserve the feeding vessels to the medial facet of the talus that is just underneath the deep deltoid ligament. Any scar tissue has to be removed. The release is sufficient when the ankle opens up symmetrically on the lateral and medial sides under axial distraction. If required, superficial deltoid fibers can also be released.[20] It is helpful to excise the tip of the medial malleolus in order to get a clear view of the span of the tibial insertion of the ligament and allow the release of the ligament in a more proximal point. Excision of the tip of the medial malleolus can minimize the risk of damage to the medial talar feeding vessels.

Lateral Gutter

Lateral ankle gutter impingement pain is less common than the medial gutter impingement. It shares similar causes of medial gutter impingement, such as a technical error of malpositioning of the prosthesis, oversizing of the prosthesis, loosening of the prosthesis, inadequate to no prophylactic gutter resection, failure to address the hindfoot malalignment, and heterotopic bone formation. Oversized tibial components usually lead to painful impingement with the fibula.[20] If the impingement is limited, bone resection at the impingement area can be considered. If the impingement is more pronounced, the component should be repositioned or replaced by a smaller one.[20] Calcaneofibular impingement can occur in cases of persistent valgus hindfoot deformity after TAR. It is also more common after TAR in varus osteoarthrosis of the ankle.[22] In cases of combined medial and lateral gutter impingement, besides oversizing the prosthetic components, especially the talar prosthesis, one should consider the possibility of subsidence of the prosthesis as a cause.[18] This subsidence should be treated by TAR revision rather than arthroscopic debridement.

Anterior Gutter

Pathologic conditions at the anterior gutter after TAR was seldom reported in the literature, although anterior ossifications had been reported and were more frequent in the Ankle Evolutive System (Transysteme-JMT Implants, Nimes, France) and HINTEGRA implants.[23] The radiological appearance of anterior ossifications may not associate with the clinical symptoms.[24]

Posterior Gutter

Heterotopic ossification occurs most commonly in the posterior gutter.[24] Posterior tibial ossifications were more frequent with the HINTEGRA Ankle Prosthesis and Salto Mobile prosthesis.[23] It was thought to be caused by a lack of posterior covering of the tibia by an inappropriately small tibial component resulting in exposure of cancellous bone posteriorly.[23] It can present as posterior ankle pain and limited ankle plantar flexion and dorsiflexion.[24] However, the occurrence of heterotopic ossification may not correlate with clinical symptoms even if there is evidence of radiologic posterior impingement. Arthroscopic resection is only indicated when there are corresponding symptoms.

Anterior Ankle Arthroscopy

The primary indication of anterior ankle arthroscopy is persistent symptomatic soft tissue and/or osseous medial and/or lateral gutter impingement. Preoperative standing radiographs or computed tomography (CT) is used to demonstrate the prosthesis-malleolar or prosthesis-hypertrophic boney contact.[12] Soft-tissue gutter impingement can present as pain in an otherwise uncomplicated TAR with clinical presentation of swelling, tenderness and pain on exertion with no identifiable cause on plain radiographs.[21] An arthroscopic procedure is contraindicated if there are complications that require revision TAR such as aseptic osteolysis and loosening, dislocation, or deep periprosthetic infection.[21]

Arthroscopic debridement has multiple potential advantages over open arthrotomy, such as a shorter recovery period, faster return to function, and less chance of deep periprosthetic infection[12,13] which is especially important for the presence of a prosthesis.

The aim of arthroscopic debridement is adequate debridement of the malleolar gutters without too much bone resection resulting in risk of destabilization of the prosthesis or periprosthetic fracture.[12,13,19,20] Whenever feasible, the debrided osseous surfaces should be sealed with bone wax to prevent hematoma and new bone formation.[20] Any hypertrophied synovial and scar tissue at the site of the pain should also be debrided.[21] With careful attention to the relevant ankle surface anatomy during portal placement and avoidance of iatrogenic damage to the TAR components themselves, arthroscopic debridement to treat impingement can be performed via routine anterior-medial and anterior-lateral portals.[13]

Arthroscopy was undertaken with patients in a supine position, and a thigh tourniquet is applied to provide a bloodless surgical field. There is controversy whether ankle distraction is used or not.[12,13,21] A 2.7-mm or 4.0-mm, 30° angled arthroscope is introduced in turn through the standard anterior-medial and anterior-lateral portals. The ankle prostheses are highly reflective and can lead to some confusion when trying to orient the arthroscope (**Fig. 1**).[12,13] The touch sensation through the tip of the arthroscopic shaver can help the identification of the intra-articular structures and orientation of the arthroscopic view (**Fig. 2**). The debridement is started at the lateral gutter if there is bilateral gutter impingement with the talar component sandwiched between the malleoli or in cases of medial gutter impingement pain, in which the talus cannot be shifted laterally to create a safe zone for debridement of posteromedial bone and increase the risk of damage of the posterior tibial neurovascular bundle. In cases when the prosthesis is wedged between both malleoli making it difficult to get any initial separation within the joint, ankle traction may be helpful to get a space at the malleolar tip for beginning of bone resection. After creating space within the lateral gutter, the arthroscope can be taken over the top of the talar component to look into the gutter

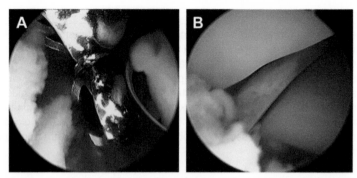

Fig. 1. Arthroscopic view from the anterior-lateral portal of an Agility TAR talar prosthesis with the shaver to the top and the mirror-image reflection to the bottom (*A*) as well as the UHMWPE insert at the top and reflection to the bottom (*B*).

(**Fig. 3**). A 70° angled arthroscope is often helpful at this point. From this anterior-to-posterior view, the talar shelf of bone or the malleolar bone within the lateral or medial gutter can be visualized as a cause of impingement and then removed (**Fig. 4**). During the bone resection, care should be taken to ensure that the blunt end of the shaver or burr with the hood is immediately adjacent to the talus to avoid excessive bone resection, which increases the risk of fracture and destabilization of the prosthesis.[12,13] Moreover, this can prevent damage to the metal and UHMWPE of the TAR implant itself. Scuffs and scratches on the metal prosthesis and UHMWPE insert can be

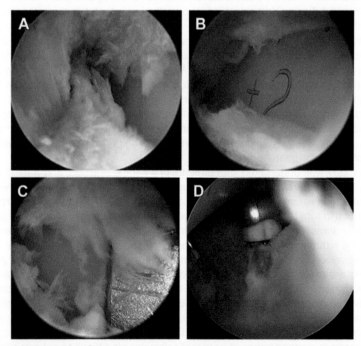

Fig. 2. Arthroscopic view from the anterior-lateral portal of the anterior-central aspect (*A*) of an Agility TAR +2 UHMWPE insert (*B*). Note the extensive scar formation engulfing the prosthetic components. The lateral tibial side is identified (*C*) followed by debridement of the lateral gutter (*D*).

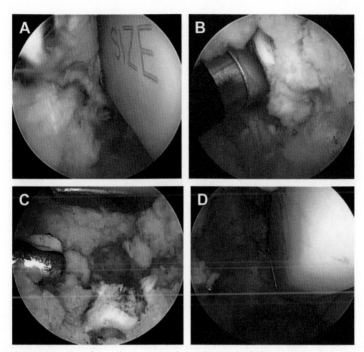

Fig. 3. Arthroscopic view from the anterior-lateral portal of the anterior-central aspect (*A*) of an Agility TAR demonstrating the extensive scar tissue formation filling the medial gutter (*B*). Following extensive debridement, the inferior part of the medial tibial sidewall can be identified (*top*) (*C*). Debridement is continued until the entire soft tissue scar is excised, thereby reducing soft tissue impingement (*D*).

documented (**Fig. 5**).[12,13] The lateral gutter is debrided with the shaver, burr, and curettes until a clear path is seen between the prosthesis and lateral malleolus. Once most of the bone has been removed from the malleolus, the remaining shelf of posterior bone can be penetrated with a drill bit, which is less likely to injure the soft tissue posteriorly than a burr.[12,13] To ensure adequate decompression, visualization of the peroneal tendons is essential after debridement on the lateral side. Similarly, visualization of the posterior tibial tendon is seen on the medial side. Intraoperative fluoroscopy is used to verify adequate debridement of all areas of osseous impingement and can be used to evaluate the amount of bone resected.[12,13]

Kurup and Taylor[19] first reported that one patient after TAR underwent arthroscopic debridement of scar tissue and impinging bone that gave good symptomatic relief. Shirzad and colleagues[13] described the details of the arthroscopic technique and reported good pain relief in 11 patients diagnosed with impingement following TAR who underwent arthroscopic decompression. Richardson and colleagues[12] reported a series of 20 ankles in 20 patients treated with arthroscopic gutter debridement, and 18 (90%) of them had sufficient follow-up. Sixteen patients (80%) reported an initial resolution of their pain following the procedure. Of these 16 patients, 6 (37.5%) developed recurrent symptoms and ultimately required further intervention.[12]

Posterior Ankle Arthroscopy/Posterior Ankle Endoscopy

The posterior arthroscopic procedure is indicated for soft tissue and/or osseous impingement of the posterior gutter and limited ankle motion. It is contraindicated in

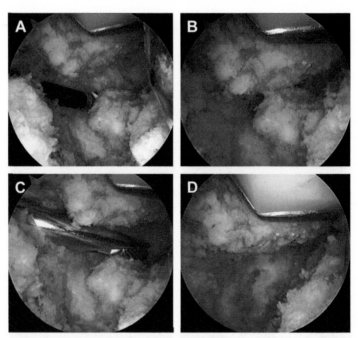

Fig. 4. Arthroscopic view from the anterior-lateral portal of the medial gutter of an Agility TAR demonstrating an exostosis off the medial talar body adjacent to the talar component (*A*) that directly abuts the medial malleolus with inversion of the ankle (*B*). An acromionizer is demonstrated before (*C*) resection of the exostosis that resolves the osseous impingement (*D*).

cases of limited ankle motion as a result of improper positioning of the prosthesis in the sagittal plane or subsidence of its component.[18,25]

Posterior ankle arthroscopy can be used in cases of soft tissue impingement. It is especially useful if concomitant anterior ankle arthroscopy is indicated, such as debridement of the medial and/or lateral gutter. This procedure can avoid change of position during the operation and minimize the risk of infection.[15,16] The posteromedial portal is just anterior to the posterior tibial tendon, and the posterolateral portal is just

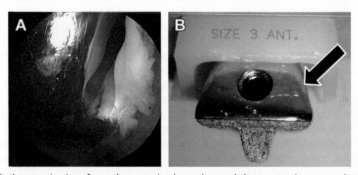

Fig. 5. Arthroscopic view from the anterior-lateral portal demonstrating extensive scratching and gouging of the dorsal-lateral surface of an Agility TAR talar component (*A*). The same talar component following explantation confirming the extensive scratching and gouging of the talar surface (*black arrow*) (*B*). Note the corresponding indentations within the UHMWPE insert.

posterior to the peroneal tendons.[15] In cases of dense scar tissue in the posterior gutter, forceful introduction into the posterior ankle gutter will cause damage to the metallic components and/or UHMWPE insert. This damage can be solved by making a larger posteromedial incision and incising the deep part of the posterior tibial tendon sheath. The space between the flexor hallucis longus (FHL) tendon and the posterior ankle capsule is developed with a hemostat. The arthroscope and shaver are inserted into this space, and arthroscopic debridement is performed anteriorly. If there is a bare bone area at the tibial plafond that is not covered by the tibial component, the debridement should be started here until the posterior edge of the tibial component baseplate is reached. The shaver should then be turned so that the debridement continues with the blunt end of the shaver touching the posterior surface of the UHMWPE liner. With the debridement going distally along the surface of the liner, the shaver will drop into the posterior ankle joint proper. The debridement is continued with the blunt end of the shaver touching the metallic talar component.

In cases of heterotopic bone in the posterior ankle gutter or limited ankle motion, the posterior ankle endoscopy[14] with patients in the prone position is preferred. Sometimes the ectopic bone can obscure the arthroscopic view, and the posterior ankle joint line cannot be assessed arthroscopically. Intraoperative fluoroscopy is useful to identify the edge of the ectopic bone, and the bone can be removed with a Kerrison rongeur (Integra, Plainsboro, NJ, USA).

In cases of ankle stiffness after TAR, the usual limitation is in dorsiflexion.[26] If persistent restriction remains in ankle dorsiflexion after gastrocnemius recession or tendo-Achilles lengthening, the next step should be posterior ankle capsulectomy, debridement of posterior ankle gutter, and release of the deep posterior deltoid ligament and the posterior talofibular ligament.[26]

Arthroscopic approach to the posteromedial ankle corner during the resection of the posteromedial ectopic bone[24] or release of the deep posterior deltoid ligament has a potential risk to the neurovascular structures. This risk will not be eliminated by instrumentation at the lateral side of the FHL tendon, as the tendon needs to be pushed medially in order to reach the posteromedial ankle corner. The displaced FHL tendon can compress on the neurovascular bundle by itself, which can be solved by slinging the FHL tendon and pulling it laterally to expose the posteromedial corner of the ankle. Another solution is to use the posterior-lateral portal as the instrumentation portal. A 70° angled arthroscope through the standard posteromedial portal or a 30° angled arthroscope through the modified posteromedial portal (1.5 cm to 2.0 cm above the standard posteromedial portal) can be used to visualize the procedure.

Procedures of the Tibia and Talus with Close Proximity to the Nonarticular Parts of the Total Ankle Replacement

The arthroscopic procedures and the lesions that are dealt within this group can affect the stability of the TAR. Periprosthetic osteolysis and cyst formation can progress without symptoms until catastrophic structural failure, mechanical loosening of the prosthesis components, or subsidence of TAR occurs. Sometimes some cysts becomes symptomatic without any evidence of collapse once a certain size has been achieved, which may be because of pressure changes of the joint fluid within the cyst.[20]

The principal cause is the osteolysis triggered by UHMWPE wear particles. However, there are polyethylene-free bone cysts that should be a result of other causes. One of the possible mechanisms is similar to that of development of a bone cyst in an osteochondral lesion. The exposed subchondral bone that is not covered by the prosthesis to the intra-articular fluid could eventually lead to a sort of synovial inclusion or cystic formation by the intra-articular synovial liquid that is under pressure in a much smaller joint than the hip or knee.[27] Preexisting subchondral cysts that are growing and disease-specific cysts (ie, rheumatoid arthritis, hemochromatosis, and so forth) are other possible causes of cysts that are not wear induced.[20]

The true extent of lucencies or cysts is often difficult to assess on plain-film radiographs and may further be obscured by the prosthetic components, particularly one that caps the talar dome. CT is superior to radiographs in detecting cysts, especially the talar ones. It can also assess the size, configuration of the cyst, and its relationship to the prosthesis, which is important in the planning of surgery.[6,18,27,28]

Signs of cyst progression on serial surveillance imaging should prompt surgical intervention.[18,29] Surgical options are curettage and autogenous or allogenic impaction bone grafting of the cyst, with and without UHMWPE insert exchange (indirect approach) or metal component revision with bone graft (direct approach through the articular part of the talus or tibia).[6,18,27,29,30] UHMWPE insert exchange is not always necessary as the cyst may not be related to wear of the liner. Loosened component or subsidence of the prosthesis indicating revision TAR favors the direct approach. If the components of the TAR can be preserved, an indirect approach is indicated. Endoscopic curettage and impaction bone grafting is a variation of the indirect approach and is particularly useful in cases of compromise of the soft tissue envelope. Moreover, the endoscopic approach may be more acceptable to patients, especially for those with an asymptomatic cyst. Contraindications for endoscopic curettage and bone grafting include the significant loss of bone stock in the tibia and/or talus, erosion and fracture of either malleolus, the presence of avascular necrosis of the talar dome, uncontained defects, and infection cysts. It is also contraindicated in the presence of loosening or subsidence of the metallic prosthetic components, significant malalignment or UHMWPE insert wear that requires exchange of the insert, or metallic component revision TAR.

Detailed preoperative surgical planning with the information from CT is the key to success. In contrast to the bone cyst associated with osteochondral lesion, the transosteochondral lesion portals are not available in the periprosthetic cysts.[31] Moreover, the posterior talar bone window posterior to the talar component can be very narrow and may not be feasible for posterior talar bone endoscopy. Anterior talar bone endoscopy portals at the talar neck are more feasible. The procedure starts with the anterior ankle arthroscopy. The UHMWPE liner should be examined for any excessive wear, and the talar and tibial components should be probed for any loosening despite a stable radiographic appearance. It should be converted to an open procedure if indicated. After examination of the components of TAR, the intra-articular scar tissue around the talar portal sites is debrided in case of talar bone cysts. In order to reach the talar dome, the anterior bone portals should be made plantar to the equator of the talar neck. It is best suited for the anterior cyst. However, for the talar dome or posterior cysts, the long portal tract from the bone portal to the cyst will hinder the freedom of the instruments. This difficulty can be partly solved by making a larger bone tunnel or using a smaller-sized arthroscope. These techniques bear the risk of iatrogenic fracture of the talar neck or breakage of the instruments. Portals at the medial and lateral talar facets anterior to the malleoli can also be used. The intramedullary components of the TAR, such as the tibial stem and screws, and the locations of the cysts at different zones of the TAR[27,28] can affect the choice of the portals. The portals should be away from the important structures, such as the neurovascular bundle, and should be through the thin cortex of the cyst and as coaxial as possible. The tibial portals should be at the level of the proximal end of the cyst in order to avoid further weakening of support to the tibial component. In order to avoid multiple attempts of drilling into the cyst and weakening the support to the tibial and talar prosthesis, intraoperative fluoroscopy or CT is needed for the establishment of the osseous portal tracts. Finally, it is important to fill all bone defects under the weight-bearing surface of the tibial base plate with impacted bone grafting.[18] Impacted bone grafting and the small bone portals can prevent the bone graft from falling into the joint and becoming loose bodies.

PROCEDURES THAT ARE AWAY FROM THE TOTAL ANKLE REPLACEMENT
Posterior Tibial Tendon Endoscopic Decompression

Soft tissue impingement can rarely occur in cases of oversized tibial component. It is usually located posteromedially affecting the flexor tendons and tibial nerve. If the tibial nerve is involved, the impinging component always needs to be repositioned or replaced.[20] If only the tibialis posterior tendonitis is present, surgical decompression of the tendon can be performed.[19] Posterior tibial tendoscopy[32] can be performed, and the medial malleolar groove is deepened anterior-medially so that the tendon can shift away from the prosthesis. The tendon sheath should be preserved in order to avoid subluxation of the tendon. The tibial component should be exchanged or repositioned if the impingement cannot be relieved. The degenerative tears of the tendon are debrided.

Endoscopic Curettage and Bone Grafting of the Fibular Bone Cyst

Bone cysts can be found in bone distant to the articulating surface of the TAR, such as the distal fibula.[33,34] Bone endoscopy with the portals at the diagonals of the cyst can be used for curettage and bone grafting. This procedure is contraindicated in cases when cortical breakage is present and plating is required or exchange of the UHMWPE liner is indicated.[33]

Endoscopic Gastrocnemius Release

As discussed earlier, gastrocnemius recession or tendo-Achilles lengthening is the first step of surgical management of limited ankle dorsiflexion after TAR. Great care must be exercised when considering whether to lengthen the Achilles. Leaving patients with a plantar flexion contracture after TAR causes abnormal gait and possibly can lead to increased midfoot stress and arthrosis with time. Distal Achilles lengthening will increase dorsiflexion but at a risk of causing push-off weakness during gait. Without proper push-off strength, the terminal plantar flexion that usually occurs will be lost resulting in a gait pattern that resembles the gait of a patient who had ankle fusion. The theoretic advantage of selective gastrocnemius lengthening is that it can increase the range of motion while not causing significant plantar flexion strength deficits. It also results in less loss of muscle bulk and contour to the lower leg compared with tendo-Achilles lengthening. Endoscopic gastrocnemius release can be either at the gastrocnemius aponeurosis distal to the gastrocnemius muscle attachment or at the intramuscular portion of the gastrocnemius aponeurosis with the uni-portal or 2-portals technique.[35–37]

Arthroscopic Subtalar or Midtarsal Arthroscopic Debridement; Arthroscopic Subtalar or Triple Arthrodesis

Despite being lower than after arthrodesis, progression to foot arthritis after arthroplasty is reported to occur in up to 15% of the cases.[21,30] Arthroscopic debridement or arthrodesis of the affected joints[10,38,39] can be performed depending on the degree of arthritic changes. The varus hindfoot deformity can be corrected during the arthroscopic subtalar arthrodesis by the closing-wedge procedure.[10,40] After correction of the varus deformity, the lateral gutter should be examined for any calcaneofibular impingement. Endoscopic lateral calcaneal ostectomy can be performed if indicated.[10,11]

Endoscopic Lateral Calcaneal Decompression

Calcaneofibular impingement can occur in cases of persistent valgus hindfoot deformity after TAR or after correction of varus hindfoot by arthroscopic subtalar arthrodesis. Lateral calcaneal ostectomy can be performed with the 2-portals or 3-portals techniques.[11,41]

Endoscopic Collateral Ligaments Repair or Reconstruction

Recently many techniques of endoscopic collateral ligament repair or reconstruction have been developed. Although open ligamentous repair or Bröstrom-Gould lateral ankle stabilization has been shown to be effective in the management of ankle instability after TAR, the efficacy of endoscopic approaches is in doubt. Most of the endoscopic techniques involve insertion of suture anchors or making bone tunnels in the lateral malleolus that would already be thinned during TAR. These techniques can cause iatrogenic fracture of the lateral malleolus. Moreover, making of the bone tunnel at the talar insertion of the anterior tibiofibular ligament may be blocked by the screw fixation in HINTEGRA Ankle Prosthesis. Finally, exchange of a larger UHMWPE liner is frequently required.[42] The surgeon should have detailed assessment and planning before considering this procedure.

SUMMARY

Foot and ankle arthroscopy and endoscopy have many potential applications to manage complications after TAR. Unfortunately there is no large-scale study to show their efficacy and safety, and the procedures should be used with caution. Additionally, these remain master arthroscopist procedures and should be performed by foot and ankle surgeons who perform them with regularity. Finally, careful evaluation and analysis of patients' problems and detailed surgical planning with appropriate combination of arthroscopic and open procedures is the key to success.

REFERENCES

1. Guyer AJ, Richardson EG. Current concept review: total ankle arthroplasty. Foot Ankle Int 2008;29:256–64.
2. Krause FG, Windolf M, Bora B, et al. Impact of complications in total ankle replacement and ankle arthrodesis analyzed with a validated outcome measurement. J Bone Joint Surg Am 2011;93:830–9.
3. Noelle S, Egidy CC, Cross MB, et al. Complication rates after total ankle arthroplasty in one hundred consecutive prostheses. Int Orthop 2013;37:1789–94.
4. Schweitzer KM Jr, Adams SB Jr, Viens NA, et al. Early prospective clinical results of a modern fixed-bearing total ankle arthroplasty. J Bone Joint Surg Am 2013;95: 1002–111.
5. Glazebrook MA, Arsenault K, Dunbar M. Evidence-based classification of complications in total ankle arthroplasty. Foot Ankle Int 2009;30:945–9.
6. Easley ME, Adams SB Jr, Hembree C, et al. Results of total ankle arthroplasty. J Bone Joint Surg Am 2011;93:1455–68.
7. Sadoghi P, Roush G, Kastner N, et al. Failure modes for total ankle arthroplasty: a statistical analysis of the Norwegian Arthroplasty Register. Arch Orthop Trauma Surg 2014;134:1361–8.

8. Gadd RJ, Barwick TW, Paling E, et al. Assessment of a three-grade classification of complications in total ankle replacement. Foot Ankle Int 2014;35:434–7.

9. Barg A, Suter T, Zwicky L, et al. Medial pain syndrome in patients with total ankle replacement. Orthopade 2011;40:991–9.

10. Lui TH, Chan KB. Arthroscopic management of late complications of calcaneal fractures. Knee Surg Sports Traumatol Arthrosc 2013;21:1293–9.

11. Lui TH. Endoscopic lateral calcaneal ostectomy for calcaneofibular impingement. Arch Orthop Trauma Surg 2007;127:265–7.

12. Richardson AB, DeOrio JK, Parekh SG. Arthroscopic debridement: effective treatment for impingement after total ankle arthroplasty. Curr Rev Musculoskelet Med 2012;5:171–5.

13. Shirzad K, Viens NA, DeOrio JK. Arthroscopic treatment of impingement after total ankle arthroplasty: technique tip. Foot Ankle Int 2011;32:727–9.

14. van Dijk CN, Scholten PE, Krips RA. 2-Portal endoscopic approach for diagnosis and treatment of posterior ankle pathology. Arthroscopy 2000;16:871–6.

15. Lui TH. Arthroscopic treatment of posterior ankle impingement in the supine position using coaxial posterior portals. Foot Ankle Int 2014;35:834–7.

16. Acevedo JI, Busch MT, Ganey TM, et al. Coaxial portals for posterior ankle arthroscopy: an anatomical study with clinical correlation on 29 patients. Arthroscopy 2000;16:836–42.

17. Schuberth JM, Babu NS, Richey JM, et al. Gutter impingement after total ankle arthroplasty. Foot Ankle Int 2013;34:329–37.

18. Jonck JH, Myerson MS. Revision total ankle replacement. Foot Ankle 2012;17: 687–706.

19. Kurup HV, Taylor GR. Medial impingement after ankle replacement. Int Orthop 2008;32:243–6.

20. Rippstein PF, Huber M, Naal FD. Management of specific complications related to total ankle arthroplasty. Foot Ankle Clin 2012;17:707–17.

21. Kim BS, Choi WJ, Kim J, et al. Residual pain due to soft-tissue impingement after uncomplicated total ankle replacement. Bone Joint J 2013;95:378–83.

22. Trajkovski T, Pinsker E, Cadden A, et al. Outcomes of ankle arthroplasty with pre-operative coronal-plane varus deformity of 10° or greater. J Bone Joint Surg Am 2013;95:1382–8.

23. Preyssasa P, Toullecc E, Henryd M, et al. Total ankle arthroplasty-three-component total ankle arthroplasty in western France: a radiographic study. Orthop Traumatol Surg Res 2012;98:S31–40.

24. Lee KB, Cho YJ, Park JK, et al. Heterotopic ossification after primary total ankle arthroplasty. J Bone Joint Surg Am 2011;93:751–8.

25. Barg A, Elsner A, Anderson AE, et al. The effect of three-component total ankle replacement malalignment on clinical outcome: pain relief and functional outcome in 317 consecutive patients. Bone Joint Surg Am 2011;93:1969–78.

26. Gérard R, Unno-Veith F, Fasel J, et al. The effect of collateral ligament release on ankle dorsiflexion: an anatomical study. Foot Ankle Surg 2011;17:193–6.

27. Rodriguez D, Bevernage BD, Maldague P, et al. Medium term follow-up of the AES ankle prosthesis: high rate of asymptomatic osteolysis. Foot Ankle Surg 2010;16:54–60.

28. Besse JL, Lienhart C, Fessy MH. Outcomes following cyst curettage and bone grafting for the management of periprosthetic cystic evolution after AES total ankle replacement. Clin Podiatr Med Surg 2013;30:157–70.

29. DiDomenico LA, Williams K. Revisional total ankle arthroplasty because of a large tibial bone cyst. J Foot Ankle Surg 2008;47:453–6.

30. Rodrigues-Pinto R, Muras J, Oliva XM, et al. Functional results and complication analysis after total ankle replacement. Early to medium-term results from a Portuguese and Spanish prospective multicentric study. Foot Ankle Surg 2013;19: 222–8.

31. Lui TH. Endoscopic curettage and bone grafting of huge talar bone cyst with preservation of cartilaginous surfaces: surgical planning. Foot Ankle Surg 2014;20(4):248–52.

32. van Dijk CN, Kort N, Scholten PE. Tendoscopy of the posterior tibial tendon. Arthroscopy 1997;13:692–8.

33. Harris NJ, Brooke BT, Sturdee S. A wear debris cyst following STAR total ankle replacement-surgical management. Foot Ankle Surg 2009;15:43–5.

34. Conti SF, Wong YS. Complications of total ankle replacement. Clin Orthop Relat Res 2001;391:105–14.

35. Saxena A, Widtfeldt A. Endoscopic gastrocnemius recession: preliminary report on 18 cases. J Foot Ankle Surg 2004;43:302–6.

36. Schweinberger MH, Roukis TS. Surgical correction of soft-tissue ankle equinus contracture. Clin Podiatr Med Surg 2008;25:571–85.

37. Lui TH. Modified endoscopic release of gastrocnemius aponeurosis. J Foot Ankle Surg 2015;54(1):140–2.

38. Lui TH. New technique of arthroscopic triple arthrodesis. Arthroscopy 2006;22: 464.e1–5.

39. Oloff L, Schulhofer SD, Fanton G, et al. Arthroscopy of the calcaneocuboid and talonavicular joints. J Foot Ankle Surg 1996;35:101–8.

40. Lui TH. Case report: correction of neglected clubfoot deformity by arthroscopic assisted triple arthrodesis. Arch Orthop Trauma Surg 2010;130:1007–11.

41. Bauer T, Deranlot J, Hardy P. Endoscopic treatment of calcaneo-fibular impingement. Knee Surg Sports Traumatol Arthrosc 2011;19:131–6.

42. Roselló Añón A, Martinez Garrido I, Cervera Deval J, et al. Total ankle replacement in patients with end-stage ankle osteoarthritis: clinical results and kinetic gait analysis. Foot Ankle Surg 2014;20:195–200.

Painful Osteophytes, Ectopic Bone, and Pain in the Malleolar Gutters Following Total Ankle Replacement

Management and Strategies

Benjamin D. Overley Jr, DPM[a],*, Thomas C. Beideman, DPM[b]

KEYWORDS

- Ankle arthroscopy • Débridement • Heterotrophic bone • Malleolar impingement
- Total ankle arthroplasty

KEY POINTS

- Osseous overgrowths leading to osteophytes and ectopic bone formation are fairly common occurrences after primary total ankle replacement.
- The most common site for ectopic bone formation is the posterior ankle joint followed by the medial and/or lateral gutters.
- Most osteophytes and ectopic bone formation do not require surgical intervention.
- When ectopic bone formation in the malleolar gutters restricts motion or is a source of pain it may require surgical intervention.
- Open and arthroscopic procedures have been described to address these postoperative complications with good relief obtained in most instances; however, a high reoperation rate exists, especially if talar component subsidence is responsible for the ectopic bone formation within the medial and/or lateral gutters.

INTRODUCTION

The incidence of osseous overgrowth after primary total ankle replacement (TAR) has been reported to range from 3.8% to 82%, but has not been linked to one clear causative entity. Lee and colleagues[1] conducted a study on 88 ankles following primary TAR and reported that 25% of patients developed ectopic bone growth. Specifically, 35% of these patients displayed bone formation at the posterior-medial and posterior-lateral quadrants of the ankle; 25% displayed only posterior-medial bone

[a] PMSI Division of Orthopedics, 1601 Medical Drive, Pottstown, PA 19464, USA; [b] Mercy Suburban Hospital, 2701 DeKalb Pike, Norristown, PA 19401, USA
* Corresponding author.
E-mail address: BOverley@pmsiforlife.com

Clin Podiatr Med Surg 32 (2015) 509–516
http://dx.doi.org/10.1016/j.cpm.2015.06.013
0891-8422/15/$ – see front matter © 2015 Elsevier Inc. All rights reserved.

formation; 25% displayed only posterior-lateral bone formation; 10% displayed anterior-medial and posterior-lateral bone formation; and 5% developed anterior-lateral and posterior-medial bone formation.[1] It is important to note that each of the patients with ectopic bone formation had some degree of posterior bone formation that is consistent with other reports following TAR.[2–5] Lee and colleagues[1] also reported that only 10% of patients who developed ectopic bone ossification were symptomatic with only 2.3% of their patients requiring surgical resection. This finding is consistent with what is reported in existing orthopedic literature relative to hip and knee replacements, with symptomatic ectopic bone ossifications resulting in severe functional loss only accounting for 1% to 2% of patients.[6]

There exists a divide in the current foot and ankle literature in this area, as many studies suggest that osteophytes and ectopic ossifications are linked to anterior and posterior impingement syndromes[4] with associated functional disabilities, such as pain with traversing uneven terrain, incline ambulation, or rising from a seated position. In contrast, other investigators do not associate a loss of function or postoperative pain with ectopic ossifications in TAR.[1,3,5,7,8]

Orthopedic data pertaining to ectopic ossification after knee and hip replacement have stirred similar critical evaluation following TAR. Early attempts to identify factors that lead to, or even predispose a patient to postoperative formation of osteophytes and/or ectopic bone ossifications are currently being conducted. It has been suggested that age, body weight (ie, increased body mass index), presence of preoperative osteophytes, and increased preoperative serum calcium and alkaline phosphatase will increase the likelihood of postoperative osteophytes and ectopic ossification in hip and knee replacements.[1,2,9] Choi and Lee[7] investigated the aforementioned predisposing factors in a series of 90 ankles following primary TAR and found that the only associated risk factor for postoperative osteophytes and ectopic bone formation was gender. Specifically, they found that men were twice as likely to develop osteophytes and ectopic ossifications as women.[7]

Other theories suggest that the formation of osteophytes and ectopic bone ossification could be a result of procedural factors as opposed to the previously discussed patient demographics. Potential factors that have been studied include the large amount of soft tissue dissection associated with the procedure, the amount of osseous trauma involved in the procedure, persistence of bone debris in the surgical field, postoperative hematoma, appropriate sizing of prosthetic components, and position of the prosthetic components leading to changes in the biomechanical axis of the ankle joint.[2] Removal of the posterior portion of the resected tibia is often difficult due to the attachment of the posterior capsular tissues and dissection occurring from the anterior aspect of the ankle for most TAR systems available in the United States. Multiple attempts at removing this portion of the tibia frequently result in morcelization of fragments. San Giovanni and colleagues[3] suggest that these morcelized portions of bone are not always completed resected and may lead to postoperative osteophytes or ectopic bone formation.

King and colleagues[2] noted that a high percentage of patients in their study with posterior osseous overgrowth had their prosthetic components inserted at an angle that was not perpendicular to the anatomic axis of the tibia, usually placed in varus or valgus with a positive slope (ie, apex posterior). They found a positive correlation between increased slope of the tibial component and uncovering of the posterior distal tibia. With decreased tibial coverage, there was found to be an increase in ectopic bone formation around the tibial tray, thus making size selection of prosthetic components and accurate insertion critical.[2] Surgeons choosing larger tibial component size to increase the amount of cortical coverage may do so at the cost of greater bone resection medially and laterally at the malleoli that can lead to malleolar fractures.

Studies have indicated that prolonged surgery time has been associated with increased ectopic bone formation as a result of increased osseous bleeding and inflammation at the surgical site.[1] In an attempt to decrease postoperative inflammation, D'Lima and colleagues[10] studied the use of prophylactic nonsteroidal anti-inflammatory drugs (NSAIDs), particularly indomethacin, and showed that it reduced the incidence of ectopic bone ossification after hip replacement. Valderrabano and colleagues[4] performed a similar study evaluating NSAID use following primary TAR; however, 63% of their patients developed ectopic ossifications despite prophylactic NSAID use.

It can be deduced by the data previously discussed that osteophytes and ectopic bone formation are frequent occurrences after primary TAR but are not always associated with painful impingement or restricted range of motion (ROM). Minimizing the rate of occurrence and/or severity of ectopic bone formation can be achieved by certain operative techniques that will be discussed, as well as strategies for managing these complications. The following will also detail procedures of choice when reoperation cannot be avoided.

DIAGNOSIS

Diagnosis of osteophytes and ectopic bone ossification is relatively straightforward, with standard radiographs showing radiodense ossifications in the ankle joint capsule, ligament attachment sites, or medial/lateral gutters (**Fig. 1**). Although visualization of these ossifications may be simple to ascertain radiographically, there may be several concurrent painful sites in the same ankle and the relevance of the ossifications identified that may be causing pain or impeding motion may be unclear. Accordingly, a detailed history is essential to a successful diagnosis. Patients will typically relate a decrease in ROM with an increase in pain compared with their initial postoperative ROM values. This can be seen at any time during the postoperative course and can occur as soon as 3 months

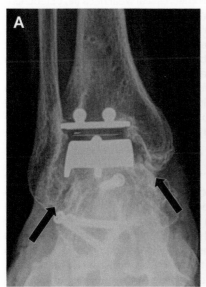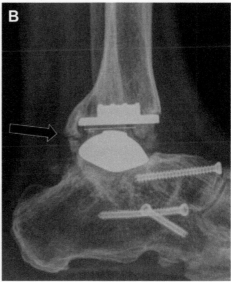

Fig. 1. Anterior-posterior (A) and lateral (B) weight-bearing radiographs 1-year postoperative demonstrating ectopic bone ossification within the medial and lateral gutters, as well as posterior ankle (*straight arrows*). This patient had very little ROM to the ankle as a result of the global ectopic bone formation engulfing this primary total ankle replacement.

postoperatively. A thorough physical examination is extremely beneficial as a diagnostic tool, including palpation of the joint lines, and gutters will usually reveal to the examiner which of these ossification sites may be the culprit. Palpation with attempted rotation, motion in the sagittal and coronal planes may also assist in determination of the causative impingement with pain in the anterior-lateral region of the lateral gutter exhibiting pain with forced dorsiflexion. More detailed diagnostic studies, such as computed tomography (CT) or single-photon emission CT scans may be beneficial in delineating impingement sites of ectopic ossification, especially in the medial and lateral ankle gutters where talar component scatter artifact from standard CT may hide or distort the osseous impingement.

The presentation of osseous versus synovial impingement as it pertains to malleolar gutter impingement may also be difficult to delineate from a clinical or radiographic study perspective. However, it should be noted that the presence of both is usually encountered during débridement and may certainly be, if not always, coexistent in malleolar gutter impingement syndromes. Injections of these regions as a diagnosis tool may also provide pertinent diagnostic information but should be used judiciously because of the risk of prosthesis contamination and deep periprosthetic infection.

A careful and honest appraisal of the implant placement and sizing may show that due to lack of bone coverage or conversely "overstuffing" the joint may be the causative factor (**Fig. 2**). Once a diagnosis is made, there are several considerations to the surgical management of these conditions and questions that require answering before proceeding with débridement. The prosthesis must be assessed critically to determine if there is loosening, subsidence, incorrect implant sizing, inadequate polyethylene insert size with lack of gutter expansion and prosthesis, or bone infection present.

If any of the causative factors are present, then a simple débridement of the offending bone and synovium will not address the underlying index cause. In cases of chronic talar subsidence, especially with talar components that may have sacrificed talar blood supply or if the prosthesis was placed in a position of biomechanical weakness (ie, osteochondral defect, fracture line, or cyst), the talus slowly depresses from axial load, which expands the medial and lateral walls of the talus that may shower the gutters with particulate osseous debris or expand into the respective malleoli causing impingement and restricted motion. In essence, the ectopic bone formations in the malleolar gutters are from talus depression and medial lateral expansion (**Fig. 3**). In all of these cases, careful considerations of polyethylene insert exchange, component exchange, or complete removal should be entertained concomitantly with the osseous débridement. If the prosthesis is stable, in acceptable alignment, and no clinical infection is present as per diagnostic studies, the next area of focus is surgical débridement of the ectopic bone.

SURGICAL TECHNIQUE

Arthroscopic débridement of painful osteophytes, ectopic bone, and soft tissue impingement in the malleolar gutters are addressed elsewhere in this issue and accordingly we focus on the open approach for these syndromes. In general, the open approach is relatively straightforward with incision planning focused to the areas of concern. Care should be taken to avoid neurovascular structures and tendons in close proximity to the planned incision, as they may be adhered to the ectopic bone or enmeshed in soft tissue scar. Acute awareness of the proximity of the polyethylene and articulating metallic prosthetic components is also essential to avoid inadvertent TAR damage.

The procedure starts with proper location of the offending region of ectopic bone and adhesive synovial tissues (**Fig. 4**). Once the soft tissues are mobilized and the

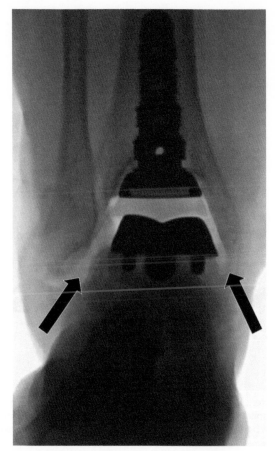

Fig. 2. Anterior-posterior image intensification view demonstrating complete talar dome coverage without overlap of the prosthetic component into the medial or lateral gutters that have also undergone through débridement (*straight arrows*).

ectopic bone circumferentially exposed, a small-diameter high-speed rotary burr is used to perform bone removal. In addition to being efficient, a secondary benefit of the thermal effect created with the use of the rotary burr is that is may discourage the reformation of the ectopic bone. Débridement may also be undertaken with bone rongeurs, sharp curettes, or osteotomes with usage of an electrocautery device to cauterize the exposed cancellous bone substrate. Application of absorbable bone wax may also help seal the cancellous bone substrate, thereby limiting osseous regeneration and recurrence of the ectopic bone.

POSTOPERATIVE CARE

The patient is typically placed in a bulky compressive dressing and is encouraged to bear weight as soon as tolerated. The only exception is if the anterior approach incision must be used, and then care must be taken to not disrupt the incision for minimum of 2 to 3 weeks. Once the incisions have healed, early active physical therapy should be undertaken with emphasis on ROM, traction, massage, and gait training.

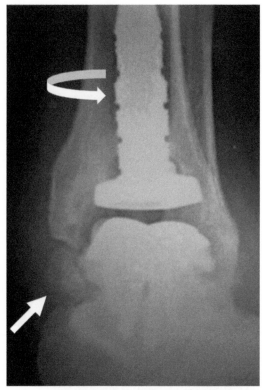

Fig. 3. Anterior-posterior radiographs 2-year postoperative demonstrating lucency surrounding the tibial component (*curved arrow*) suggestive of component loosening, as well as large medial gutter ectopic bone formation (*straight arrow*) as a result of talar component subsidence.

OUTCOMES

Shirzad and colleagues[11] described an arthroscopic technique to resect soft-tissue and osseous impingement and reported good pain relief in 11 patients. Similarly, Richardson and colleagues[12] described arthroscopic gutter débridement in a series of 20 ankles (20 patients) with 18 (90%) of them having sufficient follow-up. Sixteen patients (80%) reported an initial resolution of their pain after the procedure. Unfortunately, of these 16 patients, 6 (37.5%) developed recurrent symptoms and ultimately required further intervention likely due to talar component subsidence as the cause that required revision rather than gutter débridement.[12] Schuberth and colleagues[13] performed a retrospective review of 489 TARs using 4 different prosthetic devices, and determined that symptomatic gutter disease occurred in 34 (7%) of 489 cases. Interestingly, there was only a 2% incidence of gutter disease in the 194 ankles that had prophylactic gutter resection at the time of implantation compared with a 7% incidence in the 295 ankles that did not have gutter resection at the time of implantation. Postoperative outcomes were favorable in the 27 patients who did not have another procedure after the initial gutter débridement; however, 7 patients (21%) required reoperation following gutter débridement. The investigators concluded that prophylactic gutter resection should be considered at the time of implantation to reduce the incidence of postoperative symptoms and that although most patients had favorable outcomes after gutter débridement, there was a high reoperation rate.

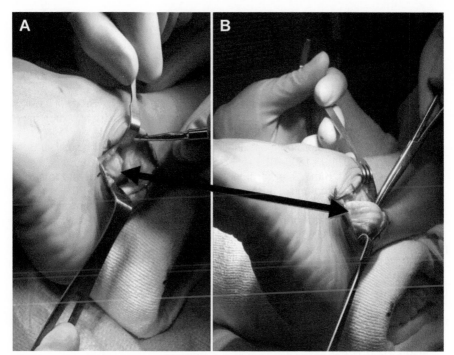

Fig. 4. Intraoperative photograph demonstrating a large laterally based ectopic bone formation (*A*) before resection, as well as attenuation of the peroneal tendons from chronic irritation about the ectopic bone (*B*).

SUMMARY

TAR is being performed more frequently around the world and accordingly an increase in complications associated with this procedure is inevitable and is being closely evaluated. The formation of osteophytes and ectopic bone peripherally around a TAR may be inevitable postoperative findings. However, as the data suggest, the appearance of these particular postoperative findings does not always equate to the need for further surgery. Open and arthroscopic approaches to address those instances in which the osteophytes and ectopic bone has slowly restricted the prosthesis ROM or are causing impingement pain are successful at resolving these complaints in most patients; however, a high reoperation rate exists, especially if talar component subsidence is responsible for the bone formation.

ACKNOWLEDGMENTS

The authors thank Bethany Worobey, MS, who assisted in the compilation and editing of this article.

REFERENCES

1. Lee KB, Cho YJ, Park JK, et al. Heterotopic ossification after primary total ankle arthroplasty. J Bone Joint Surg Am 2011;93:751–8.
2. King CM, Schuberth JM, Christensen JC, et al. Relationship to alignment and tibial cortical coverage to hypertrophic bone formation in Salto Talaris total ankle arthroplasty. J Foot Ankle Surg 2013;52:355–9.

3. San Giovanni TP, Keblish DJ, Thomas WH, et al. Eight year results of a minimally constrained total ankle arthroplasty. Foot Ankle Int 2006;27:418–26.

4. Valderrabano V, Hintermann B, Dick W. Scandinavian total ankle replacement: a 3.7 year average follow-up of 65 patients. Clin Orthop Relat Res 2004;424:47–56.

5. Wood PL, Deakin S. Total ankle replacement: the results of 200 ankles. J Bone Joint Surg Br 2003;85:334–41.

6. Berry DJ, Garvin KL, Lee S. Hip and pelvis: reconstruction. In: Beaty JH, editor. Orthopaedic knowledge update 6. Vol 39. Rosemont, IL: American Academy of Orthopedic Surgeons; 1999. p. 455–92.

7. Choi WJ, Lee JW. Heterotopic ossifications after total ankle arthroplasty. J Bone Joint Surg Br 2011;93:1508–12.

8. Kim BS, Choi WJ, Kim YS, et al. Total ankle replacement in moderate to severe varus deformity of the ankle. J Bone Joint Surg Br 2009;91:1183–90.

9. Kjaersgaard-Anderson P, Pedersen P, Kristensen SS, et al. Serum alkaline phosphatase as an indicator of heterotopic bone formation following total hip arthroplasty. Clin Orthop 1988;234:102–9.

10. D'Lima DD, Venn-Watson EJ, Tripuraneni P, et al. Indomethacin versus radiation therapy for heterotopic ossification after hip arthroplasty. J Arthrop 1989;4: 125–31.

11. Shirzad K, Viens NA, DeOrio JK. Arthroscopic treatment of impingement after total ankle arthroplasty: technique tip. Foot Ankle Int 2011;32:727–9.

12. Richardson AB, DeOrio JK, Parekh SG. Arthroscopic debridement: effective treatment for impingement after total ankle arthroplasty. Curr Rev Musculoskelet Med 2012;5:171–5.

13. Schuberth JM, Babu NS, Richey JM, et al. Gutter impingement after total ankle arthroplasty. Foot Ankle Int 2013;34:329–37.

Use of Soft-Tissue Procedures for Managing Varus and Valgus Malalignment with Total Ankle Replacement

CrossMark

Thomas S. Roukis, DPM, PhD[a],*, Andrew D. Elliott, DPM, JD[b]

KEYWORDS

- Ankle malalignment • Complications • Deformity • Musculotendinous imbalance
- Total ankle arthroplasty

KEY POINTS

- Restoring frontal plane alignment of the ankle joint during the index prosthesis surgery is essential for total ankle replacement (TAR) success.
- It is difficult to achieve frontal plane alignment during TAR through periarticular osteotomy alone.
- Tendon lengthening, ligament release, ligament reinforcement, tendon transfer, and nonanatomic tendon transfer ligament reconstructions in combination with selective use of periarticular osteotomies provides the ability to correct a variety of malalignments.
- The approach to frontal plane deformities during primary and revision TAR requires a step-wise use approach.

INTRODUCTION

Achieving a plantigrade foot and ankle is essential for the success of total ankle replacement (TAR).[1–6] Correcting osseous malalignment and soft-tissue contractures at the level of the ankle joint or distally in the foot during primary or revision TAR surgery does this. Failure to do so will lead to the phenomenon known as edge loading. Edge loading is an asymmetric loading force that affects the ultra–high-molecular-weight polyethylene insert and, indirectly, the prosthesis–bone interface causing uneven and

Financial Disclosure: None reported.
Conflict of Interest: None reported.
[a] Orthopaedic Center, Gundersen Health System, Mail Stop: CO2-006, 1900 South Avenue, La Crosse, WI 54601, USA; [b] Gundersen Medical Foundation, 1900 South Avenue, La Crosse, WI 54601, USA
* Corresponding author.
E-mail address: tsroukis@gundersenhealth.org

increased ultra–high-molecular-weight polyethylene insert wear. Edge loading increases the risk of prosthetic component aseptic loosening and eventual TAR failure.[1–3,5,6]

Henricson and Ågren[1] published a study of 196 second-generation TARs and reported that, of the ankles with preoperative varus or valgus deformities, approximately 50% (29/55 varus and 23/46 valgus) retained some malalignment after the procedure. Those retaining 15° of frontal plane deformity after the index TAR surgery had a significant increase in failure rates.[1] That study, and most other studies,[2–6] found the predominate frontal plane deformity to be ankle varus and stated that any deformity should be corrected at the time of the index TAR surgery with standard osseous cuts and soft-tissue release/reconstruction.

Soft-tissue balancing is thought to be crucial, even in ankles with unusually large coronal plane deformities. Hobson and colleagues[2] examined 91 TARs with 10° or less of frontal plane deformity and 32 TARs with frontal plane deformity between 11° and 30°. A series of osseous and soft-tissue procedures were performed to achieve hindfoot alignment to within 5° of neutral during the index surgery. At a mean follow-up of 4 years, there were no differences regarding postoperative range of motion or complications with 84% of the TARs and initial frontal plane deformity between 11° and 30° achieved final hindfoot alignment to within 5° of neutral. Similarly, Queen and colleagues[5] examined 17 TARs with greater than 15° frontal plane deformity, 21 with 5° to 15° valgus, 27 with 5° to 15° varus, and 38 with neutral alignment defined as less than 5° frontal plane deformity. A series of osseous and soft-tissue procedures were performed to achieve hindfoot alignment to within 5° of neutral during the index TAR surgery. At a mean follow-up of 2 years, there were no differences regarding clinical outcomes and physical performance measures based on preoperative frontal plane deformity when postoperative alignment is restored to within 5° of neutral during the index TAR surgery. Finally, Sung and colleagues[6] examined 20 TARs with frontal plane deformities of at least 20° and 79 ankles with deformities of less than 20°, the investigators showed no difference between the outcomes measured between these groups at 2 years postoperative. Each of these studies credited not only osseous correction, but also careful attention to soft-tissue balancing during the index TAR to ensure that the entire foot and ankle were in proper alignment as key to the success with frontal plane deformities of up to 30°.[2,5,6]

Correction of frontal plane malalignment at the time of TAR has traditionally involved a sequence of procedures that mirror each other. The general tenet of soft-tissue balancing involves the release of the contracted soft-tissue on the concave side and reinforcement on the convex side of the ankle.[1–6] Accordingly, varus malalignment correction during primary and revision TAR involves (1) removal of periarticular osteophyte formation and debridement of the medial, lateral, and posterior gutters, (2) circumferential release of the deltoid ligament complex off the distal medial tibia/medial malleolus and/or the medial talus or lengthening osteotomy of the medial malleolus, (3) transection or fractional lengthening of the posterior tibial tendon as visualized posterior to the medial malleolus, (4) correction of pedal deformities with dorsiflexory first metatarsal osteotomy and lateralizing calcaneal osteotomy, and (5) lateral ankle ligamentous plication and/or tendon transfer to reinforce lateral soft-tissue restraint.[1–9] Valgus malalignment correction during primary and revision TAR involves (1) removal of periarticular osteophyte formation and debridement of the medial, lateral, and posterior gutters, (2) circumferential release of the lateral ligament complex off the distal fibula or lengthening osteotomy of the lateral malleolus, (3) correction of pedal deformities with lateralizing calcaneal osteotomy or medial column, isolated or combined midfoot/hindfoot arthrodesis, and (5) deltoid ligament plication and/or tendon transfer to reinforce medial soft-tissue restraint.[2–7,10–12]

In addition to, and in most instances instead of, these osseous and soft-tissue procedures we have used 3 simple and reproducible soft-tissue procedures to correct varus contracture and 1 to correct valgus contracture at the time of primary or revision TAR surgery. All of these procedures can be performed using the traditional patient positioning (supine) and surgical site preparation (from the digits to above the knee) for TAR. The procedures all require additional, although minor, incisions on the operative leg and should be performed at the final stage of malalignment correction.

FLEXOR RETINACULUM RELEASE (TARSAL TUNNEL DECOMPRESSION) FOR BALANCING VARUS ANKLE CONTRACTURE DURING TOTAL ANKLE REPLACEMENT

As stated, the physician performing TAR will most often encounter a varus ankle deformity.[8,13,14] A common pathologic finding with varus ankle deformities is tethering of the hindfoot into varus owing to contracture of the deltoid ligament complex.[8,14] The deltoid ligament complex is the main restraint against valgus tilting of the talus and calcaneus and has 2 major subdivisions, the superficial and deep components.[15–17] The deep deltoid ligament layer consists of the deep anterior and posterior tibiotalar ligaments. The superficial deltoid ligament layer is more involved and consists of tibiospring, tibionavicular, tibiocalcaneal, and superficial tibiotalar ligaments.[15–17] The flexor retinaculum is continuous with most of the bands or fibers of the superficial deltoid ligament layer and, as such, can also tether the hindfoot in varus even after sequential release of the deep deltoid off of its osseous origin(s) and/or insertion(s). In these situations, we elect to perform flexor retinaculum release, which is commonly referred to as tarsal tunnel decompression. We use the anatomic landmarks for incision site mapping as described by Cortez Bezerra and colleagues.[18] First, when viewing the medial aspect of the foot and ankle, a line is drawn bisecting the medial malleolus and extended onto the sole of the foot (**Fig. 1**A, solid black line). A second line is drawn from the inferior aspect of the medial malleolus posteriorly perpendicular to the Achilles tendon (see **Fig. 1**B, solid white line). A third line is drawn from the center of the first metatarsal proximally along the medial aspect of the foot to the insertion the Achilles tendon (see **Fig. 1**C, dotted gray line). A fourth line is drawn from the middle of the inferior medial malleolus to the insertion of the Achilles tendon, thereby connecting the anterior aspect of the second line to the posterior aspect of the third line (see **Fig. 1**D, solid yellow line). The middles of the second, third, and fourth lines represent the course of the tibial neurovascular bundle nerve as they course through the tarsal tunnel and therefore ideal incision placement (see **Fig. 1**E, solid blue line). After making an incision through the skin and superficial fascia, a series of small crossed veins are encountered and these should be cauterized with bipolar cautery to limit thermal necrosis of the skin. The incision is deepened through the subcutaneous tissues where larger crossing veins are encountered and should be severed and the ends hand tied. The flexor retinaculum is then encountered. There are natural cleavage points between the flexor retinaculum and deep fascia at the proximal and distal aspects of the incision. A long, curved clamp is inserted at the natural cleavage distally and advanced proximally directly against the undersurface of the flexor retinaculum until it is brought through the proximal cleavage site. The flexor retinaculum is then transected with a scalpel in controlled fashion until all fibers are released (see **Fig. 1**F).

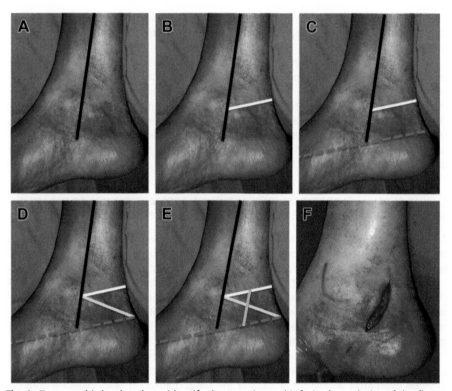

Fig. 1. Topographic landmarks to identify the superior and inferior boundaries of the flexor retinaculum and course of the neurovascular bundle as detailed in the text (*A–E*). Intraoperative photograph demonstrating complete release of the flexor retinaculum (*F*).

Unlike with the surgical treatment of tarsal tunnel syndrome, it is not routinely necessary to release the deep fascia in the lower leg or fibrous septum about the deep surface of the abductor hallucis muscle.[19,20] However, these steps may be required in severe varus ankle deformities 15° or greater when acute correction would result predictably in compression of the neurovascular components of the entire tarsal tunnel. It should be noted that the neurovascular contents of the tarsal tunnel are not actually manipulated to limit the potential for scar formation and subsequent nerve entrapment. Likewise, the skin is closed in a single layer without reapproximation of the deeper tissues to avoid compression of the neurovascular bundle.

POSTERIOR TIBIAL TENDON RECESSION FOR BALANCING VARUS ANKLE CONTRACTURE DURING TOTAL ANKLE REPLACEMENT

Traditionally, transection or fractional lengthening of the tibialis posterior tendon itself has been used to correct a varus ankle contracture.[2,3,7–9] This can be difficult to perform and unreliable. Instead of lengthening the tendon itself, the technique discussed here uses recession of the tibialis posterior tendon at the musculotendinous junction in the lower leg.[21] After the initial steps of correction are completed, the ankle is stressed in eversion and, if the ankle cannot achieve at least 5° valgus alignment with the foot maximally everted, a posterior tibial recession is performed.

The proper location for the posterior tibial recession is determined by first marking the medial aspect of the knee joint and the distal edge of the medial malleolus. Next, the medial aspect of the lower leg is divided into thirds between these 2 anatomic markers (**Fig. 2**A, dotted white lines). The incision (see **Fig. 2**A, purple line) is placed just distal to the junction of the middle and distal one-third of the lower leg directly adjacent to the posterior edge of the tibia (see **Fig. 2**A, hashed black line). The posterior tibial muscle lies directly posterior to the medial–posterior aspect of the tibia at this level in the lower leg. The incision is deepened through the subcutaneous tissues and deep fascia of the lower leg, exposing the posterior aspect of the tibia (see **Fig. 2**B). The posterior tibial muscle is easily identified directly adjacent to the posterior aspect of the tibia at this level. The posterior tibial musculotendinous junction is identified and the tendon is transected within the muscle belly with the use of electrocautery (see **Fig. 2**C) or withdrawn into the surgical field and severed with stout scissors (see **Fig. 2**D) and the foot is simultaneously dorsiflexed and everted until the varus contracture is corrected that completes the recession (see **Fig. 2**E).

MODIFIED "ALL-INSIDE" BROSTRÖM–GOULD LATERAL ANKLE STABILIZATION

Lateral ankle instability is a common cause of end-stage degenerative joint disease of the ankle and often coincides with a varus ankle deformity.[8,13,14] Most often, an open modified Broström–Gould lateral ankle stabilization is performed as a primary procedure in these situations. Recently, a technique was developed to perform an arthroscopic "all inside" modified Broström–Gould lateral ankle stabilization (Arthro-Brostrom Kit, Arthrex, Inc, Naples, FL).[22,23] We have successfully used the instrumentation that comes in this kit to aid in performing a limited dissection modified "all

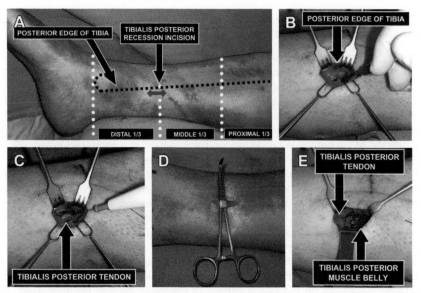

Fig. 2. Intraoperative photograph (*A*) of the medial aspect of the lower leg demonstrating the topographic anatomic landmarks used to identify the proper location for incision placement to perform posterior tibial recession. Intraoperative photograph after incision of the deep fascia exposing the posterior aspect of the tibia (*B*). The posterior tibial musculotendinous unit is exposed, and the posterior tibial tendon is isolated within the muscle itself where it is transected using electrocautery (*C*) or retrieved into the surgical field with a metallic clamp and severed with stout scissors (*D*). The completed recession is demonstrated (*E*).

inside" Broström–Gould lateral ankle stabilization. To do so, we first secure two 3-mm BioComposite SutureTak (ArthroBrostrom Kit, Arthrex, Inc) or 3.5-mm metallic cork-screw small bone anchor into the distal lateral tibia and/or fibula through the primary anterior ankle incision. The course of the inferior extensor retinaculum is marked on the skin about the anterior–lateral hindfoot/ankle and the deep capsular tissues adjacent to the lateral talar neck and anterior lateral malleolus are identified. Next, the most lateral suture strand is placed inside the Nitinol wire loop within the Curved Micro SutureLasso (ArthroBrostrom Kit, Arthrex, Inc) and passed from inside the ankle through the deep capsular tissues and out through the inferior extensor retinaculum. The next most lateral suture strand from the same anchor is then passed in similar fashion to exit the inferior retinaculum 10 mm more medial and 5 mm more distal than the first. Next, the most lateral strand from the second anchor is passed in similar fashion to exit the inferior retinaculum 10 mm more medial and 5 mm more proximal than the second suture. Finally, the most medial strand from the second anchor is passed in similar fashion to exit the inferior retinaculum 10 mm more medial and 5 mm more distal than the third suture. A 5-mm incision is placed through the skin only between the inner 2 suture strand holes and all 4 suture strands are retrieved through the central skin incision using an arthroscopic probe. The anterior–lateral soft-tissues about the hindfoot/ankle are compressed manually to bring the lateral capsule and inferior extensor retinaculum against the distal–lateral tibia/fibula. The sutures are tied under tension flush on the inferior extensor retinaculum with the ankle held in neutral position. The stability of the ankle is verified through inversion stress and anterior drawer testing under image intensification control to verify sound stabilization (**Fig. 3**).

MODIFIED EVANS PERONEUS BREVIS LATERAL ANKLE STABILIZATION FOR BALANCING VARUS ANKLE CONTRACTURE DURING TOTAL ANKLE REPLACEMENT

When modifications of the Broström–Gould lateral ankle stabilization are not sufficient, then procedures involving tendon transfer are warranted. A well-known and simple nonanatomic lateral ankle stabilization procedure was described by David L. Evans, MD, in 1953.[24] He described a release of the peroneus brevis tendon at the musculo-tendinous junction followed by retrieval at the distal end of the fibula and transfer through a drill hole in the fibula from anterior–distal to posterior–proximal followed by suturing of the peroneus brevis tendon back to itself in a shortened fashion.[24]

Explained here is a modification of the Evans peroneus brevis tendon transfer, in which the tendon is harvested through limited lateral incisions using simple topographic anatomic landmarks.[25] The harvested peroneus brevis is then transferred deep along the calcaneus and talus and secured either to the anterior–distal–lateral tibia and secured with plate and screw fixation. Although nonanatomic, this modified Evans peroneus brevis tendon transfer is useful in providing lateral ankle and subtalar stability associated with varus contractures in TAR.

For ease of harvesting the peroneus brevis tendon, proper incision placement is paramount. This is done through the following sequence of marking topographic anatomic landmarks on the lateral aspect of the lower leg and hindfoot. First, the lateral aspect of the knee joint and the distal edge of the lateral malleolus are marked. Next, the lateral aspect of the lower leg is divided into thirds between these 2 anatomic markers (**Fig. 4**A, dotted white lines). The first incision is placed just distal to midway along a line connecting the posterior–inferior tip of the lateral malleolus and superior aspect of the fifth metatarsal base (see **Fig. 4**A, yellow line). The second incision (see **Fig. 4**A, solid purple line) is placed just proximal to the junction of the middle

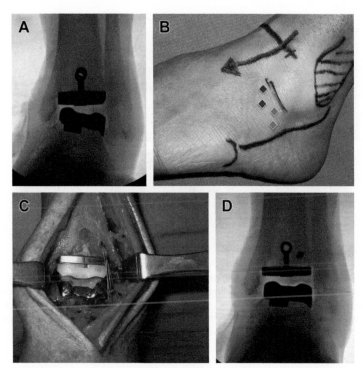

Fig. 3. (A) Intraoperative anterior–posterior image intensification inversion stress view after Salto Talaris Total Ankle Prosthesis (Tornier, Inc, Bloomington, MN) implantation demonstrating moderate persistent varus lateral ankle instability. (B) Topographic anatomy detailed in the text to identify the inferior extensor retinaculum and landmarks for the suture placement (*paired purple* and *green triangles*). (C) Location of the metallic suture anchor within the distal lateral tibia and the suture strands exiting the lateral hindfoot/ankle through the capsule and inferior extensor retinaculum. (D) Intraoperative image intensification inversion stress view after the sutures have been tied down under tension demonstrating reduction of the varus lateral ankle instability.

and distal one-thirds of the lateral aspect of the lower leg, 1 cm posterior to the posterior most edge of the fibula. The first incision is deepened through the subcutaneous tissues and peroneal retinaculum exposing the peroneus brevis superior and peroneus longus inferior (see **Fig. 4**B). The second incision is deepened through the subcutaneous tissues and deep fascia of the lower leg exposing the peroneus longus tendon, which is mobilized posteriorly thereby exposing the peroneus brevis tendon which is transected, secured with nonabsorbable suture, and freed from its extensive muscle attachments (see **Fig. 4**C). The peroneus brevis tendon is then retrieved through the distal incision and trimmed of any attached muscle fibers or loose tendon fragments in preparation for transfer (see **Fig. 4**D).

When performed concomitantly during primary or revision TAR, the peroneus brevis tendon is transferred from the lateral hindfoot incision along the calcaneus and talus into the anterior ankle incision. The ankle is held in slight eversion and the peroneus brevis tendon is secured to the distal tibia with a plate and screw construct of various configurations depending on the secondary effects afforded by the metallic fixatives (**Fig. 5**). The remnant peroneus brevis tendon is then folded over onto itself and secured with heavy gauge nonabsorbable locking sutures. In some instances, after

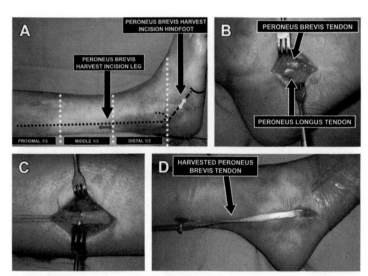

Fig. 4. Intraoperative photograph (*A*) of the lateral aspect of the lower leg demonstrating the topographic anatomic landmarks used to identify the proper location for incision placement to harvest of the peroneus brevis tendon. Intraoperative photograph demonstrating identification of the peroneus brevis tendon in the hindfoot (*B*) and lower leg (*C*) and after retrieval through the distal incision ready for transfer (*D*).

securing the tendon to the tibia, the varus ankle and lateral ankle instability are corrected but an anterior drawer remains. In these situations, the remnant peroneus brevis tendon is not folded onto itself but rather brought to the talar neck directly anterior to the talar metallic prosthetic component and secured with a plate and screw construct with the foot held at 90° to the lower leg (see **Fig. 5**F). This additional step effectively limits anterior translation of the foot. Regardless of approach, the remnant peroneus brevis tendon is then secured to the peroneus longus using multiple locked nonabsorbable sutures with the first ray in neutral to dorsiflexed position thereby correcting any first ray driven cavus foot deformity. Although not common, in situations where the Evans peroneus brevis lateral ankle stabilization procedure is deemed unnecessary but a first ray driven cavus foot is present, the peroneus brevis to peroneus longus transfer can be performed in isolation.[26]

REVERSE EVANS PERONEUS BREVIS MEDIAL ANKLE STABILIZATION FOR BALANCING VALGUS ANKLE CONTRACTURE DURING TOTAL ANKLE REPLACEMENT

Medial ankle instability secondary to deltoid ligament insufficiency is frequently encountered with end-stage degenerative joint disease of the ankle.[1,2,4–7,11,12] There are numerous procedures to correct and stabilize medial ankle instability that vary in their complexity and degree of difficulty. Although nonanatomic, this modified "reverse" Evans peroneus brevis tendon transfer provides a simple, reproducible medial ankle stabilization procedure for correction of long-standing valgus contractures during or following primary and revision TAR.[27]

Proper incision placement to harvest the peroneus brevis tendon is determined through the following sequence of topographic anatomic landmarks on the lateral aspect of the lower leg and hindfoot in the same manner as for obtained the modified Evans peroneus brevis tendon transfer noted. Next, the peroneus brevis tendon is anastomosed to the peroneus longus tendon with heavy gauge nonabsorbable suture

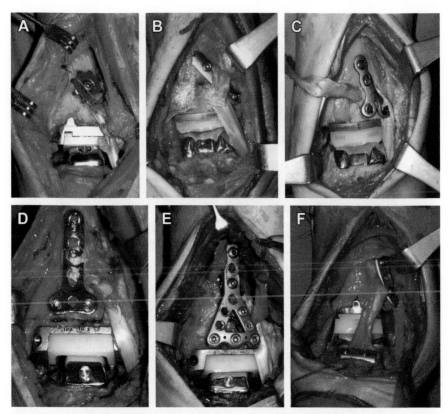

Fig. 5. Various metallic fixative constructs consist of a spiked washer and screw (*A*), oblique straight plate (*B*), Y-shaped plate (*C*), T-shaped plate (*D*), and specialty anterior tibia plate when additional support to the distal tibial component is required (*E*). The redundant peroneus brevis tendon is demonstrated as secured to the talar neck with a small plate and screw construct (*F*).

at the proximal extent of the first incision holding the first ray maximally plantarflexed and the forefoot pronated to limit any valgus thrust that could stress the deltoid ligament repair. The peroneus brevis tendon is then severed just distal to the anastomosis and secured with heavy gauge nonabsorbable sutures. The peroneus brevis tendon is then retrieved through the distal incision and trimmed of any attached muscle fibers or loose tendon fragments in preparation for transfer. The tendon is then brought through a 4-mm drill hole in the talus from lateral to medial aiming for the junction of the talar neck and body plantar to midline at the exit point medially. Sustained traction is applied to the peroneus brevis tendon for several minutes time to limit mechanical creep and subsequent loss of medial restraint. The tendon is then brought superiorly and obliquely to the anterior medial aspect of the distal tibia where it is secured under a plate and screw construct (**Fig. 6**A). Specifically, the tendon is brought under the plate from medial to lateral and then compressed between the plate and bone by tightening the screws in the plate with the tendon under maximum tension. Finally, the residual tendon is folded back onto itself and secured with multiple heavy gauge nonabsorbable sutures (see **Fig. 6**B). It is important to use intraoperative radiographic control when determining the location and path of the drill hole within the talar neck to pass the peroneus brevis tendon (see **Fig. 6**C, D).

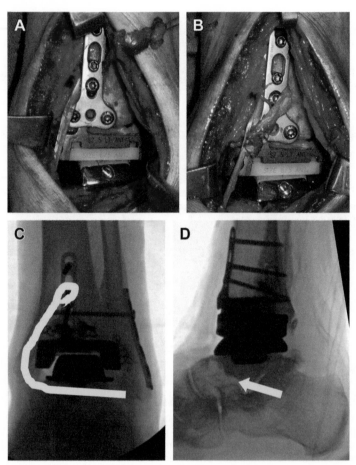

Fig. 6. The peroneus brevis tendon can be seen in the intraoperative photograph along the anterior medial aspect of the tibial component sidewall secured between the plate and distal tibia (*A*). Intraoperative photograph after completion of the peroneus brevis tendon transfer secured back onto itself demonstrating maintained anatomic alignment under valgus ankle stress (*B*). Mortise (*C*) and lateral (*D*) ankle image intensification views demonstrating the orientation of the peroneus brevis autograft (*yellow outline*) and drill hole location (*yellow arrow*).

COMPLICATIONS AND CONCERNS

The most common complications associated with release of the flexor retinaculum release and posterior tibial tendon recession are failure to achieve complete release leading to undercorrection of the varus contracture. It is recommended to always fully assess the soft-tissue flexor retinaculum to assess for complete release and, if identified as excessively taught, then the proximal and distal deep fascia segments should undergo release until no further compression of the neurovascular bundle is identified and reduction of the varus contracture is confirmed. With posterior tibial tendon recession, it is common to have several bands of tendon remain after severing the tendon and it is very important to double check after the index release to make certain no residual tendon fibers remain. Additionally, it is important to perform the procedure as described because the flexor digitorum tendon lies directly adjacent but superficial to the posterior tibial tendon at this level in the lower leg and can inadvertently be mistaken and severed. Finally, care must be taken with the index dissection and retrieval of the posterior tibial tendon because the neurovascular bundle is in close proximity and can be injured inadvertently.

The most common complications associated with the modified "all-inside" Broström–Gould lateral ankle stabilization, as well as modified Evans peroneus brevis lateral and medial ligament reconstruction, are failure to achieve appropriate stability at the time of index surgery and loss of correction during the postoperative period leading to recurrent instability. We limit the modified "all-inside" Broström–Gould lateral ankle stabilization to minor lateral ankle instability. If any doubt exists we prefer the stability of the modified Evans peroneus brevis lateral ankle stabilization to the simplicity of the modified "all-inside" Broström–Gould lateral ankle stabilization. Additionally, the modified "all-inside" Broström–Gould lateral ankle stabilization has the additional risk of injury to the lateral branch of the superficial peroneal nerve during passage of the sutures and great care must be taken to minimize this risk through proper technique. The use of secure plate and screw fixation for securing the peroneus brevis tendon to bone is superior to soft-tissue anchors and interference screws, regardless of whether a medial or lateral ankle stabilization procedure is performed. After verifying that the ankle is stable to inversion stress, it is important to check for an anterior drawer that, when present, should be corrected by securing the remnant peroneus brevis tendon to the anterior talar neck as described. With all of these procedures, careful patient selection and proper surgical technique are mandatory to achieve consistently good outcomes.

SUMMARY

When combined with established techniques for the correction of osseous malalignment and soft-tissue contracture, these described techniques offer safe, straightforward, minimally invasive, and reproducible procedures that can effectively correct frontal plane deformities resulting from end stage degenerative joint disease of the ankle. The use of reproducible topographic anatomic landmarks is essential to perform these techniques properly and limit the potential for complications. In all of these procedures, recovery is dictated by the TAR and additional ancillary procedures performed.

REFERENCES

1. Henricson A, Ågren PH. Secondary surgery after total ankle replacement, the influence of preoperative hindfoot alignment. Foot Ankle Surg 2007;13:41–4.
2. Hobson SA, Karantana A, Dhur S. Total ankle replacement in patients with significant pre-operative deformity of the hindfoot. J Bone Joint Surg Br 2009;91:481–6.
3. Kim BS, Choi WJ, Kim YS, et al. Total ankle replacement in moderate to severe varus deformity of the ankle. J Bone Joint Surg Br 2009;91:1183–90.
4. Woo JC, Yoon HS, Lee JW. Techniques for managing varus and valgus malalignment during total ankle replacement. Clin Podiatr Med Surg 2013;30:35–46.
5. Queen RM, Adams SB Jr, Viens NA, et al. Differences in outcomes following total ankle replacement in patients with neutral alignment compared with tibiotalar joint malalignment. J Bone Joint Surg Am 2013;95:1927–34.
6. Sung KS, Ahn J, Lee KH, et al. Short-term results of total ankle arthroplasty for end-stage ankle arthritis with severe varus deformity. Foot Ankle Int 2014;35: 225–31.

7. Coetzee JC. Management of varus or valgus ankle deformity with ankle replacement. Foot Ankle Clin 2008;13:509–20.

8. Mayich DJ, Daniels TR. Total ankle replacement in ankle arthritis with varus talar deformity: pathophysiology, evaluation, and management principles. Foot Ankle Clin 2012;17:127–39.

9. Redfern JC, Thordarson DB. Achilles lengthening/posterior tibial tenotomy with immediate weightbearing for patients with significant comorbidities. Foot Ankle Int 2008;29:325–8.

10. Doets HC, van der Plaat LW, Klein JP. Medial malleolar osteotomy for the correction of varus deformity during total ankle arthroplasty: results in 15 ankles. Foot Ankle Int 2008;29:171–7.

11. Brunner S, Knupp M, Hintermann B. Total ankle replacement for the valgus unstable osteoarthritic ankle. Tech Foot Ankle Surg 2010;9:165–74.

12. Brooke BT, Harris NJ, Morgan S. Fibula lengthening osteotomy to correct valgus mal-alignment following total ankle arthroplasty. Foot Ankle Surg 2012;18:144–7.

13. Thomas RH, Daniels TR. Ankle arthritis. J Bone Joint Surg Am 2003;85:923–36.

14. Saltzman CL, Salamon ML, Blanchard GM, et al. Epidemiology of ankle arthritis: report of a consecutive series of 639 patients from a tertiary orthopaedic center. Iowa Orthop J 2005;25:44–6.

15. Harper MC. Deltoid ligament: an anatomical evaluation of function. Foot Ankle 1987;8:19–22.

16. Earll M, Wayne J, Brodrick C, et al. Contribution of the deltoid ligament to ankle joint contact characteristics: a cadaver study. Foot Ankle Int 1996;17:317–24.

17. Hintermann B, Golanó P. The anatomy and function of the deltoid ligament. Tech Foot Ankle Surg 2014;13:67–72.

18. Cortez Bezerra MJ, Dias Leite JA, Neto JE, et al. Endoscopic release of the tarsal tunnel: a suggested surgical approach. Acta Ortop Bras 2005;13:46–8.

19. Heimkes B, Posel P, Stotz S, et al. The proximal and distal tarsal tunnel syndromes: an anatomical study. Int Orthop 1987;11:193–6.

20. Lau JT, Daniels TR. Tarsal tunnel syndrome: a review of the literature. Foot Ankle Int 1999;20:201–9.

21. Roukis TS. Tibialis posterior recession for balancing varus ankle contracture during total ankle replacement. J Foot Ankle Surg 2013;52:686–9.

22. Acevedo JI, Mangone PG. Arthroscopic lateral ankle ligament reconstruction. Tech Foot Ankle Surg 2011;10:111–6.

23. Cottom JM, Rigby RB. The "all inside" arthroscopic Broström procedure: a prospective study of 40 consecutive patients. J Foot Ankle Surg 2013;52:568–74.

24. Evans DL. Recurrent instability of the ankle: a method of surgical treatment. Proc R Soc Med 1953;46:343–4.

25. Roukis TS. Modified Evans peroneus brevis lateral ankle stabilization for balancing varus ankle contracture during total ankle replacement. J Foot Ankle Surg 2013;52:789–92.

26. Schweinberger MH, Roukis TS. Balancing of the transmetatarsal amputation with peroneus brevis to peroneus longus tendon transfer. J Foot Ankle Surg 2007;46:510–4.

27. Roukis TS, Prissel MA. Reverse Evans peroneus brevis medial ankle stabilization for balancing valgus ankle contracture during total ankle replacement. J Foot Ankle Surg 2014;53:497–502.

Osteotomies for Managing Varus and Valgus Malalignment with Total Ankle Replacement

Nikolaos Gougoulias, MD, PhD[a],
Nicola Maffulli, MD, MS, PhD, FRCP, FRCS (Orth)[b,c],*

KEYWORDS

- Ankle • Joint replacement • Varus • Valgus • Osteotomy

KEY POINTS

- Advances in total ankle replacement (TAR) surgery in recent years allowed expansion of indications to include deformed ankles.
- Accurate preoperative planning and individualization of the procedure, is essential. Staged procedures are sometimes needed.
- Medial malleolus, fibula, supramalleolar, calcaneus, first metatarsal and proximal tibia osteotomies, can be performed to neutrally align a TAR.
- The choice of the procedure depends on the level of the deformity (intra-articular vs extra-articular; proximal, within, or distal to, the ankle).
- Equally good outcomes to nondeformed ankles can be obtained, if the TAR is well-aligned, but only short-term results have been published.

INTRODUCTION

Given that ankle arthritis is usually posttraumatic and a result of chronic instability, coronal plane (varus more frequently than valgus) malalignment is a common feature of degenerate ankles. Significant varus or valgus alignment (>10°, according to most investigators) has been considered a risk factor for early failure, and therefore a

[a] Department of Trauma and Orthopaedics, Frimley Health NHS Foundation Trust, Frimley Park Hospital, Portsmouth Road, Camberley, Surrey GU16 7UJ, UK; [b] Department of Musculoskeletal Disorders, Faculty of Medicine and Surgery, University of Salerno, Salerno, 89100 Italy; [c] Centre for Sports and Exercise Medicine, Barts and The London School of Medicine and Dentistry, Mile End Hospital, London E1 4DG, UK
* Corresponding author. Department of Musculoskeletal Disorders, Faculty of Medicine and Surgery, University of Salerno, Salerno, 89100 Italy.
E-mail address: n.maffulli@qmul.ac.uk

Clin Podiatr Med Surg 32 (2015) 529–542
http://dx.doi.org/10.1016/j.cpm.2015.06.014
0891-8422/15/$ – see front matter © 2015 Elsevier Inc. All rights reserved.

relative contraindication for total ankle replacement (TAR).[1,2] Malalignment and imbalance of the TAR should be avoided, as it would lead to abnormal distribution of contact pressures, polyethylene wear, osteolysis, and early failure.[3–9] Some surgeons have, however, expanded the indications of TAR to include ankles with preoperative deformity of 15° or more, performing adjunctive procedures to correct coronal plane alignment and stability (eg, subtalar or triple arthrodesis, osteotomies, soft tissue releases, and ligament reconstructions).[10–26] We present the rationale, surgical techniques, and outcomes of re-alignment osteotomies that have been described (ie, medial malleolus, fibula, distal or proximal tibia, calcaneus, first metatarsal) as adjunctive procedures performing TAR for deformed ankles. This article focuses on coronal plane deformities, but one has to bear in mind that ankle deformity rarely occurs in one plane only.

GENERAL CONSIDERATIONS AND PREOPERATIVE EVALUATION

It is generally acceptable, but also evidence proven, that surgical outcomes after TAR are better in experienced hands.[27] Therefore, it is essential that the surgeon has gained enough experience performing TARs in nondeformed ankles, before extending his or her indications. Nevertheless, it is not only the surgical skills and expertise, but also patients' selection and accurate preoperative evaluation of the problem and planning of the procedure that are key issues for success when performing these demanding operations. Appropriate preoperative patient counseling, assessment of patients' comorbidities (eg, diabetes mellitus), and also of their functional needs and expectations, are important issues that can guide decisions regarding a patient's suitability for a complex TAR. In other words, "treat the patient, and not just the ankle," or "patient's selection is important." In the era of increasing incidence of litigation against surgeons, it is essential to make the patient aware of the risk of early failure of the TAR, especially if preoperative deformity is present.

Careful clinical examination is required, to assess the following:

- Condition of the skin
- Scars from possible previous operations
- Circulation and sensation in the lower leg and foot
- Alignment of the whole extremity (knee, patellofemoral joint, and hip)
- Gait pattern
- Range of movement of the ankle and the surrounding joints
- Presence of soft tissue contractures (eg, Achilles tendon, gastrocnemius muscle, deltoid ligament)
- Function of the peroneal tendons (insufficiency in varus ankles, muscle spasm in valgus ankles)
- Function of tibialis posterior tendon (tendinopathy, insufficiency in valgus ankles and feet)
- Presence of clinical deformity (static and/or dynamic)
- Possibility of ligamentous instability (lateral or medial)
- Condition of the shoes (for increased wear on the lateral/medial heel)

Appropriate imaging is, obviously, essential. Weight-bearing (WB), anteriorposterior (AP), and lateral radiographs of the ankle and foot should be obtained. The foot/ankle lateral WB view reveals how flat the foot is and helps identifying degenerative changes in the other hindfoot joints. The talocalcaneal axis and talonavicular joint congruity (affected in planovalgus feet) are checked on the foot AP WB radiograph. Ankle AP WB and mortise views may be indicative of subfibular impingement in valgus aligned feet. Oblique views of the foot will reveal the presence of anteromedial osteophytes. Most foot and ankle surgeons advocate the use of the (posteroanterior) hindfoot alignment radiograph as proposed by Saltzman and el-Khoury,[28] to assess the alignment of the hindfoot, and not of the ankle only. For patients with gross deformity, long leg standing views are needed.

Further imaging is often needed, depending on the examination findings. A computed tomography (CT) scan could reveal the details of osseous anatomy or joint degenerative changes. When CT is combined with a radionuclide bone scan (single-photon emission CT–CT), it can detect the "hot spots" that cause pain (eg, possibility of degenerative changes in the subtalar and talonavicular joints). If soft tissue abnormalities (eg, peroneal, Achilles or tibialis posterior tendinopathy, deltoid and spring ligament integrity, sinus tarsi scar tissue) are expected, an MRI scan is superior. Depending on available expertise, ultrasound scanning can be used to diagnose tendon pathology or nerve entrapment.

Before proceeding with the surgical procedure, the surgeon should be able to answer the questions shown in **Table 1**.

PRINCIPLES AND INDICATIONS FOR OSTEOTOMIES COMBINED WITH TOTAL ANKLE REPLACEMENT: GENERAL PRINCIPLES

The choice of adjuvant procedures that will aid performing a well-aligned TAR depends obviously on the answers given in the questions listed in **Table 1**. The treatment has to be individualized, as one procedure does not fit all situations encountered. One simple rule to remember is to perform the osteotomy at the level where the deformity has developed, and to treat the cause of the deformity (eg, proximal, at, or distal to, the ankle joint).

If the subtalar and/or talonavicular joints are arthritic and painful, arthrodesis of these joints, sometimes also involving the calcaneocuboid joint (triple arthrodesis) is

Table 1
Questions for the surgeon planning a complex TAR

Question	Answer Given by
Do the possible benefits of performing a complex total ankle replacement outweigh the risks for this particular patient?	Patient (!) Preoperative discussion
Is the ankle deformity intra-articular or extra-articular? What is the cause?	Radiographs History
What is the degree of varus/valgus deformity at the ankle joint?	Anteroposterior standing radiograph
What is the hindfoot alignment?	Saltzman view[28] Clinical examination
Is the knee joint and proximal tibia neutrally aligned?	Long leg standing view Clinical examination
Is there degeneration of the subtalar and talonavicular joints (do we need to fuse any joints)?	Radiographs Scan (computed tomography, MRI)
Is the subtalar joint mobile?	Clinical examination
Is there calf muscle/Achilles tendon contracture?	Silfverskiold test[29]
Is the cavovarus foot deformity hindfoot or forefoot driven?	Coleman block test[30]
What is the underlying pathology in valgus ankles (eg, deltoid, tibialis posterior tendon damage)?	Scan (MRI, ultrasound)

required. It is at the surgeon's discretion to perform fusion(s) as a staged procedure, or for a TAR to be performed in the same sitting. Soft tissue releases (eg, Achilles tendon lengthening) and/or ligamentous or tendon reconstructions (eg, repair of lateral ligaments, tendon transfers to reconstruct a deficient tibialis posterior tendon in valgus ankles) also may be required. In the current article, we focus on the osteotomies that can be performed to neutralize the deformed hindfoot.

We want to emphasize that the rationale of performing lower extremity osteotomies in patients with early arthritis, who do not need a TAR, is slightly different. In those cases the role of the osteotomy is to alter the WB axis of the lower leg, so as to improve the symptoms by loading a "healthy" part of the arthritic joint and postpone the need for a TAR or ankle arthrodesis. When a TAR is performed, however, the aim of adjuvant procedures together with the tibial and talar bone cuts is to produce a "perfectly neutral" alignment if possible. This is to balance a fully congruent TAR, avoiding edge loading.

EXTRA-ARTICULAR DEFORMITY

Extra-articular deformity is related to structures proximal (eg, knee and tibia), or distal (eg, heel, foot) to the ankle joint. If the patient had previously sustained a tibia fracture (distal, mid-shaft, or proximal), the deformity is likely to be extra-articular, and should be corrected with an osteotomy as close as possible to the level of the deformity, the so called CORA (center of rotation of angulation), according to the principles of deformity correction.[31] Usually it is a distal tibia fracture that will have resulted in varus or valgus ankle osteoarthritis. A supramalleolar osteotomy (SMO) may then be required.

In the presence of knee varus/valgus or rotational malalignment, a proximal tibia or a distal femoral osteotomy may be required. If tibial torsion is present (eg, as a result of a malunited tibia fracture), a rotational tibial osteotomy should be performed at the supramalleolar level. The presence of tibial torsion can be suspected from lateral position of the patella causing patella maltracking and patellofemoral joint pain.

When the varus hindfoot alignment is a result of cavovarus deformities, like the ones seen in patients with Charcot-Marie-Tooth disease, the deformity arises from the heel. In those cases, the rules of cavus foot deformity correction apply.[32] The features of cavovarus foot deformity are contracture of the Achilles tendon, heel varus, plantar flexion of the first metatarsal, peroneus brevis weakness, and tibialis posterior tightness. For those patients, a calcaneal lateralization (lateral heel shift) osteotomy is indicated, along with appropriate soft tissue procedures. If the first ray is plantarflexed and (according to the Coleman block test) the hindfoot varus is forefoot driven, a dorsal closing wedge (elevating) first metatarsal osteotomy is indicated.[32] The osteotomy helps restoring more normal first metatarsal-talus relation in the sagittal plane (**Fig. 1**). This will allow the high medial arch to drop, and will drive the hindfoot into more physiologic valgus.

INTRA-ARTICULAR DEFORMITY

When the deformity is the consequence of chronic lateral ankle instability, the talus becomes incongruent within the mortise, and gradually more cartilage is worn out on the medial half of the (varus ankle) joint. Thus, the deformity is intra-articular. Therefore it is unlikely that an extra-articular procedure can correct the deformity. In those cases, adjustment of the tibial plafond cut to correct the deformity is used, but for significant deformities this alone may not be effective in balancing the TAR. The "medial structures" need to be released. Traditionally the release involves the deltoid ligament,

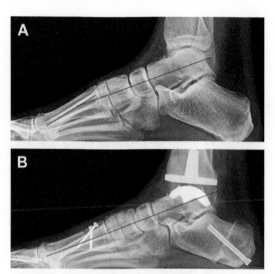

Fig. 1. Cavovarus ankle-foot deformity is characterized by heel varus, plantarflexed first metatarsal, and tight Achilles tendon (A). TAR is combined with calcaneal osteotomy (medial heel shift), and dorsal closing wedge first metatarsal osteotomy to dorsiflex the first ray. The calcaneal osteotomy is allowed to displace proximally, to functionally lengthen the Achilles tendon. The talus-first metatarsal axis in the sagittal plane is restored, and the calcaneal pitch angle is reduced (B).

but in ankles with excessive varus deformity, this may not be enough either. Thus, one has to lengthen the "medial wall" to balance the TAR. This is the rationale behind the lengthening osteotomy of the medial malleolus (**Fig. 2**).[15,16,20] One other option for larger varus deformity is the "plafondplasty," described by Ryssman and Myerson.[15] The osteotomy is guided from the supramalleolar region to the plafond, and bone graft is used to lengthen the medial wall of the ankle. It was proposed that it is performed as a staged procedure before the TAR.[15]

The common causes of valgus ankle osteoarthritis are malunion of a malleolar fracture, deltoid ligament rupture, or advanced tibialis posterior tendon dysfunction. Valgus alignment can be the result of fibula shortening/malunion after a high fibula (Weber B), pronation external rotation fracture. In those cases, a fibula-lengthening osteotomy may be indicated (**Figs. 3** and **4**).[17] Another option is to perform a supramalleolar tibia medial closing wedge osteotomy that can correct the ankle valgus alignment and effectively produce relative fibula shortening, to realign the mortise.[18]

When intra-articular ankle valgus occurs as a result of deltoid and/or spring ligament injury, a deltoid and/or spring ligament repair/reconstruction will be required. A medialization calcaneal osteotomy may help balancing the TAR (see **Fig. 3**). Realistically, patients requiring TAR, as a result of chronic medial instability, have developed subtalar joint degeneration, and the best option is probably subtalar or triple fusion in combination with TAR, rather than a joint-preserving procedure. The same applies for ankle arthritis in planovalgus feet in the advanced stages of tibialis posterior dysfunction, where triple arthrodesis is required.

Fig. 5 provides an overview and an algorithm for the management of ankle and hindfoot coronal plane malalignment in combination with TAR.

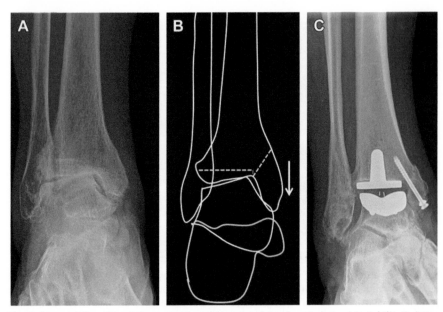

Fig. 2. Varus deformity of the arthritic ankle, related to chronic lateral instability is intra-articular (*A*). Analysis of the deformity and preoperative planning for TAR (*B*) shows that the calcaneus is neutrally aligned, and that more bone needs to be resected on the lateral tibial plafond (*yellow dotted line*). This will tighten the medial joint even further. Therefore, extensive deltoid ligament lengthening is required. Sometimes this is not sufficient and a medial malleolus lengthening osteotomy is needed (*white dotted line, white arrow*). The total ankle replacement is now neutrally aligned (*C*).

SURGICAL TECHNIQUES: GENERAL CONSIDERATIONS

As mentioned earlier, osteotomies may be performed simultaneously or as staged procedures in combination with TAR. It largely depends on the surgeon's experience and preference, but also on the length of the planned procedure. Typically these procedures are performed with a thigh tourniquet applied and inflated. One has to consider the expected duration of tourniquet inflation, and has to plan to probably release the tourniquet having to re-inflate it after sufficient time, for procedures that are expected to last for more than 2.5 hours.

When surgeries around the knee are required first (eg, high tibial or distal femoral osteotomy, knee replacement, or soft tissue reconstructions), to correct the alignment, the authors recommend for those to be performed as staged procedures, and the TAR to be performed separately. This is because of the higher risks for complications (eg, thromboembolic events, neurovascular compromise), but also because of the difficulties of rehabilitating the patient (different regimens used for knee and ankle surgeries).

The ankle/hindfoot surgery is performed with the patient in the supine position under general and/or spinal anesthetic, whereas nerve blocks can offer postoperative analgesia. Ipsilateral buttock elevation is needed to eliminate physiologic external rotation of the leg, so the ankle faces upward. The skin is sterilized above the knee, so knee and lower leg are visible to the surgical team. An image intensifier is essential, and the positioning of the machine and the screen should allow easy use for anteroposterior and lateral imaging, and viewing of the fluoro-images.

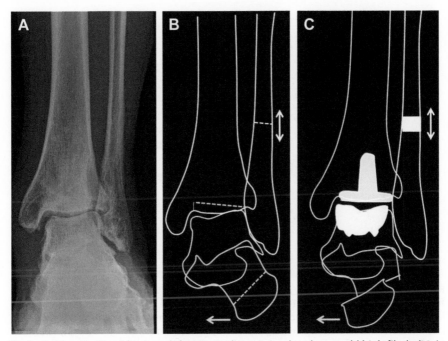

Fig. 3. Ankle arthritis and valgus deformity in this case is related to an old high fibula (Maisonneuve) fracture with syndesmosis disruption (*A*). Analysis of the deformity and preoperative planning for TAR (*B*) reveals widening of the medial clear space (between talus and medial malleolus), loss of anatomic alignment of the syndesmosis, shortening of the fibula (intra-articular deformity), and valgus heel alignment (extra-articular deformity). In such a case, TAR requires more bone resection on the medial side of the tibial plafond (*yellow dotted line*), and can be combined with fibula-lengthening osteotomy (*white dotted line, double headed arrow*), to restore anatomy of the joint. The extra-articular component of the deformity (heel valgus) would require a calcaneal varisation osteotomy (*yellow dotted line*) (*B*) and medial translation of the calcaneal tuberosity (*yellow arrow*), (*B, C*).

A 15-cm midline ankle incision and an anterior ankle approach (lateral to the extensor hallucis longus tendon sheath) are usually recommended for the vast majority of ankle prostheses. Depending on the adjunctive procedures, the incision and surgical approach may have to be extended proximally or laterally, or other incisions may be used, as well. One has to consider leaving safe distances between incisions to avoid skin perfusion compromise and wound-healing problems. If multiple incisions are needed, one may have to consider performing staged procedures.

SUPRAMALLEOLAR OSTEOTOMY

One has to plan the osteotomy preoperatively and calculate the desired displacement and correction that needs to be achieved. The level of the SMO has to take into consideration whether a stemmed tibial implant is used,[1] and the type of osteotomy fixation (eg, type of plate). Ideally, one would want to perform the osteotomy through the same anterior approach as the TAR. It is performed using a thin oscillating saw, or making multiple holes using a 2-mm drill, then connecting those using a sharp osteotome. An alternative would be the "Gigli-saw." Any effort should be made to minimize thermal bone damage to facilitate rapid healing.

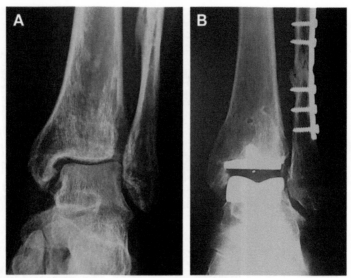

Fig. 4. In this case, ankle valgus arthritis is a result of an old Wb C fracture of the fibula. The fibula is short and rotated (*A*). The heel is, however, neutral. More tibial bone is lost on the lateral half; therefore, more bone needs to be resected on the medial tibial plafond to perform a TAR. A fibula-lengthening osteotomy is required to restore anatomy, lengthen the "lateral column" of the ankle, and neutralize TAR alignment (*B*).

In cases with abnormal tibial torsion, a rotational displacement is required. Before performing the osteotomy, 2 Kirschner wires are inserted at either side of the planned osteotomy line, at an angle equal to the rotational deformity. After the osteotomy is performed, the 2 fragments are mobilized in a way that the wires become parallel, and the fixation is performed.

When varus deformity is corrected, a medial opening or a lateral closing wedge SMO can be performed. Often (depending on the amount of correction) a fibula osteotomy, to allow displacement of the SMO, will be needed, as well. The medial opening wedge SMO is advantageous in those cases, as it does not shorten the leg, and, more importantly, it allows lengthening of the "medial wall" and effectively functional release of the tight medial structures in varus ankles. A lateral closing wedge SMO, on the other hand, is biomechanically more stable. Alternatively, a focal dome osteotomy can be performed.

The SMO can be also performed to reduce intra-articular ankle varus. However, because the level of the osteotomy is different (extra-articular) than the level of the deformity (intra-articular), residual varus can be expected. This will be corrected through the actual TAR (bone cuts and soft tissue releases).

CALCANEAL OSTEOTOMY

Calcaneal osteotomies are performed in combination with TAR for patients with cavovarus feet, heel varus, and ankle arthritis. The osteotomy is performed through either an oblique or an "L-shaped" lateral calcaneal approach. The authors prefer the "L-shaped" incision (**Fig. 6**), as it carries a smaller risk of sural nerve damage and offers excellent exposure to the calcaneal tuberosity. It is part of the extensile lateral approach used for fixation of calcaneal fractures. The calcaneus is osteotomized

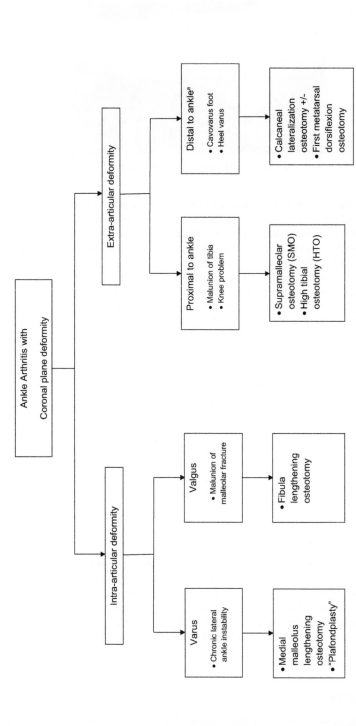

Fig. 5. Overview and algorithm for the management of ankle and hindfoot coronal plane malalignment in combination with TAR. [a] Planovalgus foot deformities with ankle arthritis usually require fusion procedures (subtalar or triple arthrodesis).

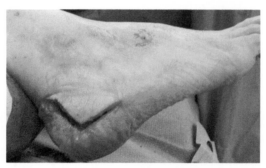

Fig. 6. Calcaneal osteotomy can be performed through a lateral "L"-shaped incision.

using an oscillating saw, perpendicular to the lateral calcaneal cortex, until the medial cortex is reached. The osteotomy is then completed using an osteotome, to avoid damage of the neurovascular bundle. A laminar spreader is used between the 2 fragments to stretch the soft tissues and facilitate lateral displacement of the calcaneal tuberosity by approximately 10 mm. Displacement of the osteotomy is easier with the knee slightly flexed (gastrocnemius relaxed). Once adequate displacement is achieved, the knee is extended for the gastrocnemius to tighten and the osteotomy to be "locked" in position. One can allow some proximal displacement of the calcaneal tuberosity to functionally lengthen the Achilles tendon. The osteotomy is easily fixed using a cannulated compression screw over a guide wire, inserted from the heel. Intraoperative image intensification is used.

FIRST METATARSAL OSTEOTOMY

The indication is forefoot-driven hindfoot varus, in cavovarus feet, identified using the Coleman block test during clinical examination. Usually a dorsal closing wedge (dorsiflexion) first metatarsal osteotomy is performed in combination with a calcaneal osteotomy (described earlier in this article). A dorsal incision at the level of the proximal half of the first metatarsal is used. A dorsal oblique wedge is excised from the proximal first metatarsal metaphysis. Care is taken to avoid fracturing the plantar cortex. A reduction forceps is used to close the osteotomy that is fixed with 2 compression screws (see **Fig. 1**).

MEDIAL MALLEOLUS OSTEOTOMY

This is indicated in excessive intra-articular varus deformities (>15°) after generous deltoid ligament release has been performed. A vertical osteotomy from the supramalleolar region down to the "shoulder" of the ankle is performed (see **Fig. 2**). The medial malleolus is moved distally until the TAR alignment is satisfactory (neutral). The osteotomy is typically fixed with 2 screws, after the final implants are inserted, although it has been originally proposed that it can be left without fixation[20]; however, this carries the risk of nonunion. Lateral ligament repair or reconstruction may be needed in those ankles at the end of the procedure.

PLAFONDPLASTY

This is a procedure proposed by Ryssman and Myerson[15] for ankle varus deformities greater than 20°, and is performed separately from the TAR. In those incongruent ankles, the medial tibial plafond is completely depleted of cartilage, has developed a groove, and the medial malleolus appears dysplastic. The osteotomy is performed starting from the supramalleolar region, aiming for the medial half of the medial plafond. Care is taken not to violate the joint, by inserting Kirschner wires. The osteotomized medial malleolus is hinged medially until most of the varus deformity is corrected, and bone graft is inserted (**Fig. 7**). The osteotomy is fixed with a plate and allowed to unite. Usually some residual varus is apparent, and this is fully corrected when a TAR is performed at a later stage.

FIBULA-LENGTHENING OSTEOTOMY

The indication is intra-articular valgus ankle malalignment, as a result of a malunited distal fibula fracture (see **Figs. 3** and **4**). This osteotomy directly addresses the cause of the deformity. The ankle was destabilized and drifted into valgus, because the "lateral wall" was shortened. A fibula osteotomy requires a direct lateral incision. A "Z" bone cut is performed and the fibula is fixed in the desired length using a dynamic compression plate. Bone graft can be used to fill in the gaps of the lengthened bone.

IMMEDIATE POSTOPERATIVE CARE

Most surgeons advocate the use of ankle immobilization in a posterior splint or removable boot for 3 weeks after a TAR for the anterior ankle wound to heal, before progressing with WB and physiotherapy. When osteotomies are performed, the immobilization and non-WB status may have to be extended for at least 6 weeks, for some osseous union to have occurred at the osteotomies. Physical and

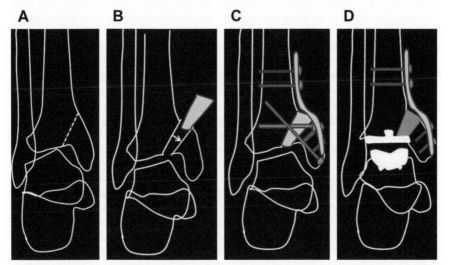

Fig. 7. In cases of excessive varus deformity and articular incongruity between tibia and talus (*A*), a staged procedure including a "plafondplasty" may be needed to restore tibiotalar joint congruity. This involves a distal tibia osteotomy through the articular surface (*white dotted line*). (*B*) The osteotomy is displaced medially (*white arrow*) to lengthen the medial column. This requires filling the gap in the distal tibia with bone graft (usually allograft). Some residual varus may be observed at this stage. Fixation is required as shown (*C*). The TAR is performed at a second stage. Tailoring the tibia bone cut will allow balancing of the TAR in neutral position in the coronal plane (*D*).

pharmacologic thromboprophylaxis is recommended for 6 weeks or until ambulatory, although published evidence is scarce and weak.

REHABILITATION AND RECOVERY

Once the wounds have healed at approximately 3 weeks postoperatively, a removable boot can be used for the patient to commence ankle range of movement exercises, remaining non-WB. Partial WB can be initiated at 6 weeks, progressing to full WB (usually this is possible after 2–3 months). Full recovery is expected a year postoperatively, but may take longer.

CLINICAL RESULTS IN THE LITERATURE

Several articles have described the surgical techniques[10–18] and others reported on clinical outcomes of TAR in deformed ankles.[8,9,19–26] One cannot isolate many studies reporting on outcomes of TARs combined with osteotomies, as these procedures are part of the whole spectrum of surgery performed for ankles with greater than 10° coronal plane deformity.

Doets and colleagues[20] reported on his series of 15 TARs in varus ankles, requiring a medial malleolar lengthening osteotomy. Only one TAR had failed after a follow-up period of 2 to 8 years, despite 2 malleoli that ended up with asymptomatic nonunion.

Jung and colleagues[23] reported good early results (12–43-months follow-up) in 10 ankles undergoing mobile-bearing TAR and cavus foot correction performing combined calcaneal (9 ankles) and first metatarsal osteotomies (4 ankles). The ankles were neutrally aligned postoperatively.

Interestingly, Reddy and colleagues[24] showed that preoperative varus deformity of greater than 10° in 43 ankles, treated with the Scandinavian TAR (Waldemar Link, Hamburg, Germany/Small Bone Innovations, Inc, Morrisville, PA/Stryker Orthopedics, Mahwah, NJ) were corrected with soft tissue procedures only, without performing osteotomies. However, 3 ankles with deformity greater than 25° failed.

A French study[25] reviewed the outcomes in 21 TARs with deformity of greater than 10°, all requiring additional procedures, many of which were osteotomies. Six (28%) of 21 ankles had residual postoperative deformity requiring further corrective surgery (osteotomies), whereas 3 TARs (14%) had already failed (requiring revision or fusion) at 3 years. However, the investigators had used the Ankle Evolutive System (Transysteme-JMT Implants, Nimes, France) (now withdrawn from the market because of high rates of osteolysis),[1] in 16 of their 21 ankle replacement surgeries, and this may have skewed their results.

The general impression reviewing the literature reporting on outcomes of TAR in deformed ankles, is that preoperative deformities could be corrected in more than 85% of cases when adjuvant soft tissue procedures and osteotomies were performed. Outcomes, at least in the short to medium term, were as good as for TARs performed for nondeformed ankles, if neutral postoperative alignment was achieved.[6,8,9,19,21,22,26] The evidence is scarce, however, and of moderate quality, as it is revealed only from evidence-based medicine level III or IV studies, with heterogeneity of surgical procedures performed, and generally short follow-up periods. Therefore, definite conclusions regarding the success of these complex procedures cannot be drawn.

SUMMARY

Joint replacement is an option for varus and valgus ankles, provided a balanced, neutrally aligned TAR can be performed. Accurate preoperative assessment of the deformity is essential for appropriate selection of adjuvant procedures. Osteotomies performed proximal (tibial), within (malleolar), or distal to (calcaneal, metatarsal) the ankle allow deformity correction. Outcomes can be expected to be as good as of those ankles without coronal plane malalignment, at least in the short term.

REFERENCES

1. Gougoulias N, Maffulli N. History of total ankle replacement. Clin Podiatr Med Surg 2013;30(1):1–20.
2. Benthien RA. Challenging the anxiety over coronal plane deformity: commentary on an article by Robin M. Queen, PhD, et al.: "Differences in outcomes following total ankle replacement in patients with neutral alignment compared with tibiotalar joint mal-alignment". J Bone Joint Surg Am 2013;95(21):e170.
3. Gougoulias N, Khanna A, Maffulli N. How successful are current ankle replacements? A systematic review of the literature. Clin Orthop Relat Res 2010; 468(1):199–208.
4. Saltzman CL, Tochigi Y, Rudert MJ, et al. The effect of agility ankle prosthesis misalignment on the peri-ankle ligaments. Clin Orthop Relat Res 2004;424:137–42.
5. Haskell A, Mann RA. Ankle arthroplasty with preoperative coronal plane deformity. Clin Orthop Relat Res 2004;424:98–103.
6. Wood PL, Deakin S. Total ankle replacement. The results in 200 ankles. J Bone Joint Surg Br 2003;85(3):334–41.
7. DeOrio JK, Easley ME. Total ankle arthroplasty. Instr Course Lect 2008;57: 383–413.
8. Barg A, Elsner A, Anderson AE, et al. The effect of three-component total ankle replacement malalignment on clinical outcome: pain relief and functional outcome in 317 consecutive patients. J Bone Joint Surg Am 2011;93(21):1969–78.
9. Barg A, Knupp M, Henninger HB, et al. Total ankle replacement using HINTE-GRA, an unconstrained, three-component system: surgical technique and pitfalls. Foot Ankle Clin 2012;17(4):607–35.
10. Choi WJ, Yoon HS, Lee JW. Techniques for managing varus and valgus malalignment during total ankle replacement. Clin Podiatr Med Surg 2013;30(1):35–46.
11. Coetzee JC. Surgical strategies: lateral ligament reconstruction as part of the management of varus ankle deformity with ankle replacement. Foot Ankle Int 2010;31(3):267–74.
12. DeOrio JK. Peritalar symposium: total ankle replacements with malaligned ankles: osteotomies performed simultaneously with TAA. Foot Ankle Int 2012; 33(4):344–6.
13. Mann HA, Filippi J, Myerson MS. Intra-articular opening medial tibial wedge osteotomy (plafond-plasty) for the treatment of intra-articular varus ankle arthritis and instability. Foot Ankle Int 2012;33(4):255–61.
14. Mayich DJ, Daniels TR. Total ankle replacement in ankle arthritis with varus talar deformity: pathophysiology, evaluation, and management principles. Foot Ankle Clin 2012;17(1):127–39.
15. Ryssman DB, Myerson MS. Total ankle arthroplasty: management of varus deformity at the ankle. Foot Ankle Int 2012;33(4):347–54.
16. Tan KJ, Myerson MS. Planning correction of the varus ankle deformity with ankle replacement. Foot Ankle Clin 2012;17(1):103–15.
17. Brooke BT, Harris NJ, Morgan S. Fibula lengthening osteotomy to correct valgus mal-alignment following total ankle arthroplasty. Foot Ankle Surg 2012;18(2): 144–7.

18. Barg A, Pagenstert GI, Leumann AG, et al. Treatment of the arthritic valgus ankle. Foot Ankle Clin 2012;17(4):647–63.
19. Hobson SA, Karantana A, Dhar S. Total ankle replacement in patients with significant pre-operative deformity of the hindfoot. J Bone Joint Surg Br 2009;91(4): 481–6.
20. Doets CH, van der Plaat LW, Klein JP. Medial malleolar osteotomy for the correction of varus deformity during total ankle arthroplasty: results in 15 ankles. Foot Ankle Int 2008;29(2):171–7.
21. Kim BS, Choi WJ, Kim YS, et al. Total ankle replacement in moderate to severe varus deformity of the ankle. J Bone Joint Surg Br 2009;91(9):1183–90.
22. Queen RM, Adams SB Jr, Viens NA, et al. Differences in outcomes following total ankle replacement in patients with neutral alignment compared with tibiotalar joint malalignment. J Bone Joint Surg Am 2013;95(21):1927–34.
23. Jung HG, Jeon SH, Kim TH, et al. Total ankle arthroplasty with combined calcaneal and metatarsal osteotomies for treatment of ankle osteoarthritis with accompanying cavovarus deformities: early results. Foot Ankle Int 2013;34(1):140–7.
24. Reddy SC, Mann JA, Mann RA, et al. Correction of moderate to severe coronal plane deformity with the STAR ankle prosthesis. Foot Ankle Int 2011;32(7): 659–64.
25. Trincat S, Kouyoumdjian P, Asencio G. Total ankle arthroplasty and coronal plane deformities. Orthop Traumatol Surg Res 2012;98(1):75–84.
26. Trajkovski T, Pinsker E, Cadden A, et al. Outcomes of ankle arthroplasty with pre-operative coronal-plane varus deformity of 10° or greater. J Bone Joint Surg Am 2013;95(15):1382–8.
27. Henricson A, Nilsson JÅ, Carlsson A. 10-year survival of total ankle arthroplasties: a report on 780 cases from the Swedish Ankle Register. Acta Orthop 2011;82: 655–9.
28. Saltzman CL, el-Khoury GY. The hindfoot alignment view. Foot Ankle Int 1995; 16(9):572–6.
29. Singh D. Nils Silfverskiöld (1888-1957) and gastrocnemius contracture. Foot Ankle Surg 2013;19(2):135–8.
30. Deben SE, Pomeroy GC. Subtle cavus foot: diagnosis and management. J Am Acad Orthop Surg 2014;22(8):512–20.
31. Lamm BM, Paley D. Deformity correction planning for hindfoot, ankle, and lower limb. Clin Podiatr Med Surg 2004;21(3):305–26.
32. Ortiz C, Wagner E, Keller A. Cavovarus foot reconstruction. Foot Ankle Clin 2009; 14(3):471–87.

Management of Osseous and Soft-Tissue Ankle Equinus During Total Ankle Replacement

Thomas S. Roukis, DPM, PhD*, Devin C. Simonson, DPM

KEYWORDS

- Arthroplasty - Complications - Fixed bearing polyethylene insert - Prosthesis
- Surgery

KEY POINTS

- At the time of total ankle replacement, correction of osseous equinus involves anterior tibiotalar cheilectomy and correction of soft-tissue ankle equinus involves either tendo-Achilles lengthening or gastrocnemius recession.
- After joint resection for the specific total ankle replacement system used, the posterior ankle capsule and deep crural fascia are resected followed in more severe deformities by release of the posterior portions of the medial and lateral collateral ligament complexes.
- Ankle dorsiflexion is primarily controlled and restricted not by a single structure but rather by the interaction between most of the ankle ligaments and posterior periarticular capsule structures.
- Further research on this topic is required as combined osseous and soft-tissue ankle equinus is infrequently encountered and more meaningful data are needed to help guide treatment.

INTRODUCTION

Obtaining functional alignment of a total ankle replacement, including physiologic sagittal plane range of motion, is paramount for a successful outcome.[1–9] Soft-tissue ankle equinus correction with either tendo-Achilles lengthening or gastrocnemius recession and posterior ankle capsule release and, in more significant contractures, medial and lateral collateral ligament complex release after osseous joint

Financial Disclosure: None reported.
Conflict of Interest: None reported.
Orthopaedic Center, Gundersen Health System, Mail Stop: CO2-006, 1900 South Avenue, La Crosse, WI 54601, USA
* Corresponding author.
E-mail address: tsroukis@gundersenhealth.org

resection, has been described to achieve physiologic sagittal plane range of motion during primary and revision total ankle replacement.[6,10–19] However, correction of severe osseous equinus has only infrequently been discussed and specifically through surgical technique description for the Agility Total Ankle Replacement Systems (DePuy Orthopaedics, Warsaw, IN, USA).[15–18,20]

LITERATURE REVIEW

Queen and colleagues[21] published a study examining the differences in outcomes between patients who underwent concomitant superficial posterior muscle compartment lengthening with total ankle replacement and those who received total ankle replacement alone. In their prospective, nonrandomized study, they examined a total of 229 patients, with 37 undergoing concomitant gastrocnemius recession, 22 undergoing concomitant triple hemisection percutaneous tendo-Achilles lengthening, and 170 undergoing total ankle replacement alone. They compared patients' preoperative status to their 1-year postoperative status with regard to patient-reported outcomes, physical performance, and lower extremity gait mechanics. They found a significant improvement in the superficial posterior muscle compartment lengthening group for most variables between the preoperative and 1-year postoperative scores and that this improvement was greater than that seen in the isolated total ankle replacement group. The investigators point to the possibility that use of concomitant superficial posterior muscle compartment lengthening with total ankle replacement can achieve better postoperative hindfoot position and thus may increase implant longevity by more closely approximating normal ankle anatomy.

DeOrio and Lewis[19] found that a Strayer-type gastrocnemius recession performed in tandem with total ankle replacement resulted in a significant and reproducible increase in dorsiflexion regardless of the results of intraoperative Silfverskiöld test on 29 consecutive patients. They highlight the preference for a gastrocnemius recession over a tendo-Achilles lengthening because of potential push-off and plantarflexion weakness with the latter.

In an anatomic study published in 2011, Gérard and colleagues[22] investigated the effect of ankle collateral ligament release on dorsiflexion, specifically following section of the posterior deep deltoid and the posterior talofibular ligament. In 18 cadaveric specimens, they found a mean increase in ankle dorsiflexion following isolated deep posterior deltoid ligament versus posterior talofibular ligament to be 7.45° versus 3.5°, respectively. They concluded that if following gastrocnemius recession or tendo-Achilles lengthening, persistent restriction remains in ankle, the next step should involve release of the deep deltoid ligament.

SURGICAL TECHNIQUE

Under general anesthesia with a popliteal and saphenous nerve blockade, an anterior ankle incision is made overlying the extensor hallucis longus tendon and the junction between this tendon laterally and the tibialis anterior tendon maintained within its sheath medially was developed and carried down to the underlying tibia and talus. Resection of scar tissue and inflamed synovium allows direct visualization of the ankle joint. Following wide resection of the global anterior ankle osteophytes and removal of any deep retained hardware, ankle dorsiflexion is usually improved but not enough to allow for total ankle replacement to proceed. Therefore, a tendo-Achilles lengthening or gastrocnemius recession is performed.[23]

For the tendo-Achilles lengthening, multiple anatomic considerations have led to the use of incisions placed at 2, 5, and 8 cm proximal to the Achilles tendon insertion as the authors' preferred method. The watershed area of the Achilles tendon is from 2 to 6 cm proximal to its insertion and is an area of relative avascularity that is highly susceptible to rupture. Incisions are placed at the extremes of the watershed area to promote healing and 3 cm apart to reduce the risk of tendon disruption. The most distal portion of the Achilles tendon is thin and narrow and therefore susceptible to rupture or transection of more than half the tendon fibers. The tendon becomes more substantial at 2 cm proximal to its insertion making this a good location for incision placement. This incision is also proximal enough to maintain the heel contour, reducing the likelihood of irritation on the heel contour of the shoe, and allows access to the plantaris tendon medially, which can be transected at this level to aid in equinus correction, if required. A #64 beaver blade is preferred to perform the procedure. An initial percutaneous stab incision is performed in a longitudinal direction at the center of the Achilles tendon 2 cm proximal to its insertion onto the calcaneus. The longitudinal incision is preferred because it does not gap when ankle dorsiflexion is performed to lengthen the tendon. The blade should advance only through the Achilles tendon proper. The blade is turned medially to transect the medial half of the tendon. A second longitudinal stab incision is made 3 cm proximal to the first with the blade turned laterally to incise the lateral half of the Achilles tendon, and then a third stab incision is made 3 cm proximal to the second for transection of the medial half of the tendon. The foot is rotated at the ankle into controlled dorsiflexion to achieve between 0° and 5° of passive ankle dorsiflexion with the knee fully extended.

For gastrocnemius recession, incision placement is determined by marking out the medial aspect of the knee joint and the distal edge of the medial malleolus. The medial aspect of the lower leg is divided into thirds between these 2 anatomic markers. To perform a Vulpius-type gastrocnemius recession, which is the authors' preferred technique, the incision is placed at the middle of the middle third of the medial aspect of the lower leg, 2 cm posterior to the posterior most edge of the medial face of the tibia. The location can be verified by palpating the medial head of the gastrocnemius muscle, with the incision located just distal to this structure. A 3-cm linear incision is made in this location, and a hemostat is placed into the incision and opened in line with the incision site. Care should be taken to avoid disruption of crossing veins that are often present traversing the incision site and can obscure the operative field. Subcutaneous adipose tissue is swept aside with a moist sponge and the surgeon's index finger. Wide retractors are placed at the edges of the incision and the deep fascia is visualized. The deep fascia is incised in line with the skin incision, exposing the underlying gastrocnemius aponeurosis that is then also incised in the same manner. A tissue elevator is passed from medial to lateral, identifying the plane between the gastrocnemius aponeurosis and deep fascia until it is palpated on the lateral side of the leg. As the elevator is removed, it is swept from distal to proximal in a windshield wiper fashion to further define this plane. A large scissor is used to transect the gastrocnemius aponeurosis from medial to lateral. The plantaris tendon is easily identified as the most medial structure within the surgical field and transected when visualized. A small portion of the remaining aponeurosis can be visualized at the anteromedial edge of the incision site and should also be transected with care taken to avoid injury to the great saphenous nerve and vein, which course in close proximity to the tibia at this level of the lower leg. The foot is rotated at the ankle into controlled dorsiflexion to achieve between 0° and 5° of passive ankle dorsiflexion with the knee fully extended, and the surgical site is inspected to make certain complete recession of the gastrocnemius aponeurosis has occurred.

Once completed, the foot can usually achieve neutral dorsiflexion but not beyond (**Fig. 1**). This movement is enough to allow the total ankle replacement bone resection

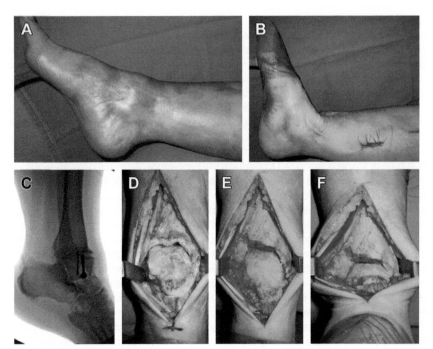

Fig. 1. Intraoperative photograph of the medial foot/lower leg demonstrating the fixed combined osseous impingement and soft-tissue contracture before (*A*) and following (*B*) correction. As demonstrated in the intraoperative lateral ankle image intensification view (*C*) and photograph (*D*), the global anterior ankle osteophytes impede dorsiflexion of the foot. After an aggressive ankle cheilectomy including hardware removal (*E*) followed by open Vulpius gastrocnemius recession, the foot can be brought to neutral position (*F*).

to proceed based on the specific prosthetic system used. Once the bone is resected, the next surgical step is a release of the passive capsuloligamentous periarticular structures. It should be noted that dorsiflexion is primarily controlled and restricted not by a single structure but rather by the interaction between most of the ankle ligaments. The periarticular soft-tissue release starts with the posterior ankle capsule, which should be excised until the posterior tibial tendon is visualized medially, the flexor hallucis longus muscle and tendon centrally, and the peroneal tendons laterally. The posterior ankle capsule excision is best accomplished with a narrow, curver osteotome used to incise the capsule adjacent to the resected bone surfaces followed by use of a pituitary rongeur to extirpate the capsule in segments. The adipose tissue within the retro-Achilles area can be removed to expose the deep crural fascia that can be released with a narrow curved osteotomy to further reduce posterior soft-tissue constraint.

The final step would be to perform release of the posterior deep deltoid ligament and then, if needed, the talofibular ankle ligament, as these ligaments provide dorsiflexion restraint (**Fig. 2**). Both these ligaments are released with a narrow curved osteotome inserted between the posterior edge of the talar body and the respective malleolus. The osteotome is advanced inferiorly and then gently twisted around the posterior edge of the respective malleolus to release the ligamentous tissues being careful not to pry on the malleolus to minimize the risk of fracture. The release is complete

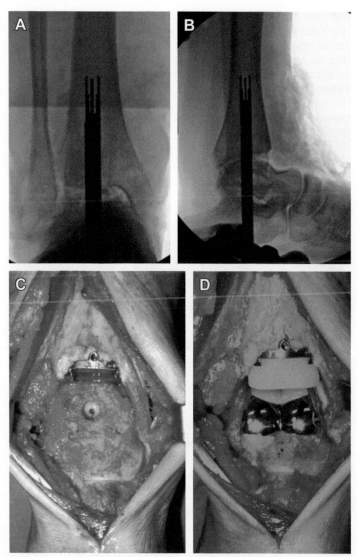

Fig. 2. Intraoperative anterior-posterior (*A*) and lateral (*B*) image intensification views after completion of the intramedullary alignment rod process within the foot holder. Intraoperative photograph after polymethylmethacrylate cement stabilization of the INBONE II Total Ankle Replacement System (Wright Medical Technologies, Inc, Memphis, TN, USA) tibial base plate and intramedullary stem components demonstrating the preserved talar body supply (*C*). The drill channels for the talar stem and 2 anterior pegs can be seen. In this instance, the posterior ankle capsule has been resected and the posterior deep deltoid ligament and talofibular ligament released. Intraoperative photograph after polymethylmethacrylate cement stabilization of the INBONE II Total Ankle Replacement System sulcus design talar component and 10-mm stem (*D*).

medially when the posterior tibial tendon can be visualized adjacent to the central portion of the medial malleolus. The release laterally is complete once the peroneal tendons can be visualized adjacent to the central portion of the lateral malleolus. Following the above-mentioned procedures, the ankle should be able to achieve full, fluid dorsiflexion and plantarflexion with no frontal plane instability appreciated on manual stress examination (**Fig. 3**).

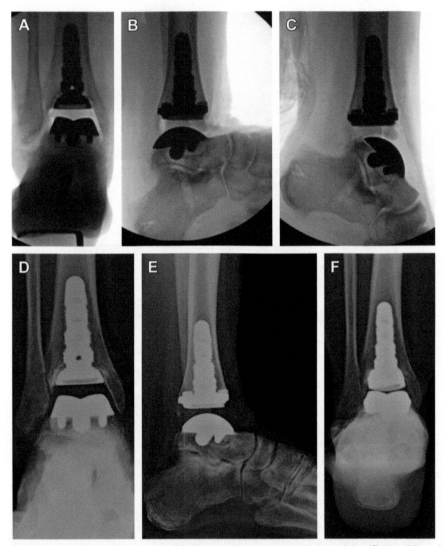

Fig. 3. Intraoperative image intensification anterior-posterior (*A*), lateral dorsiflexion (*B*), and lateral plantarflexion (*C*) views after implantation of the INBONE II Total Ankle Replacement System. Note the full sagittal plane motion achieved and maintained frontal plane stability as a result of the sulcus talar component and sulcus polyethylene insert. Anterior-posterior (*D*), lateral (*E*), and hindfoot (*F*) alignment weight bearing radiographs obtained 3.5 years after implantation of the INBONE II Total Ankle Replacement System with anterior tibiotalar joint cheilectomy, posterior superficial muscle compartment lengthening, posterior ankle capsule release, and medial and lateral collateral ligament complex fractional release.

COMPLICATIONS AND CONCERNS

The most common complications are overlengthening of the posterior muscle compartment leading to weakness and undercorrection leading to recurrent soft-tissue ankle equinus contracture. It is recommended that tendo-Achilles lengthening procedures are immobilized and the patient maintained non–weight bearing until healed followed by extensive physical therapy to improve function. In contrast, gastrocnemius recession allows for early range of motion once the anterior ankle incision has healed and weight bearing once osseous integration of the metallic components has occurred. There is also less reliance on physical therapy to restore push-off power. For these reasons, a gastrocnemius is the preferred method over tendo-Achilles lengthening for addressing soft-tissue ankle equinus whenever possible.

During resection of the posterior ankle capsule it is possible to damage the posterior medial neurovascular bundle and any of the tendons encountered. Similarly, during release of the medial and lateral ligamentous complexes it is possible to damage the adjacent tendons, fracture the malleoli, or create instability with an overzealous release. Careful patient selection and proper surgical technique are mandatory to achieve consistently good outcomes.

SUMMARY

The available literature on techniques available for correction of osseous and soft-tissue equinus at the time of index total ankle replacement is sparse. However, the combination of anterior tibiotalar joint cheilectomy, posterior superficial muscle compartment lengthening, posterior ankle capsule release, and release of the posterior portions of the medial and lateral collateral ligament complexes offers the ability to correct even the most severe deformities. Proper surgical technique when performing these procedures is imperative to minimize complications. Further research on this topic is required to help guide treatment, as the specific techniques that are most beneficial remain a matter for conjecture and the exact order to perform these procedures to achieve the best clinical outcome remains unanswered.

REFERENCES

1. Gould JS. Revision total ankle arthroplasty. Am J Orthop (Belle Mead NJ) 2005; 34:361.
2. Haddad SL, Coetzee JC, Estok R, et al. Intermediate and long-term outcomes of total ankle arthroplasty and ankle arthrodesis. J Bone Joint Surg Am 2007;89: 1899–905.
3. Guyer AJ, Richardson G. Current concepts review: total ankle arthroplasty. Foot Ankle Int 2008;29:256–64.
4. Gougoulias NE, Khanna A, Maffulli N. How successful are current ankle replacements? A systematic review of the literature. Clin Orthop Relat Res 2010;468: 199–208.
5. Easley ME, Adams SB, Hembree WC, et al. Current concepts review: results of total ankle arthroplasty. J Bone Joint Surg Am 2011;93:1455–68.
6. Roukis TS. Incidence of revision after primary implantation of the agility total ankle replacement system: a systematic review. J Foot Ankle Surg 2012;51:198–204.
7. Roukis TS. Salvage of a failed "DePuy Alvine Total Ankle Prosthesis" with Agility LP custom stemmed tibial and talar components. Clin Podiatr Med Surg 2013;30: 101–9.

8. Prissel M, Roukis TS. Incidence of revision following primary insertion of the STAR implant: a systematic review. Clin Podiatr Med Surg 2013;30:237–50.

9. Pappas MJ, Buechel Sr FF. Failure modes of current total ankle replacement systems. Clin Podiatr Med Surg 2013;30:123–43.

10. Alvine FG. Total ankle arthroplasty: new concepts and approach. Contemp Orthop 1991;22:397–403.

11. Alvine FG. The agility ankle replacement: the good and the bad. Foot Ankle Clin 2002;7:737–53.

12. Hintermann B. Complications of total ankle arthroplasty. Chapter 11. In: Hintermann B, editor. Total ankle arthroplasty: historical overview, current concepts, and future perspectives. New York: Springer; 2005. p. 163–84.

13. Myerson MS. Total ankle replacement. Chapter 24. In: Myerson MS, editor. Reconstructive foot and ankle surgery: management of complications. 2nd edition. Philadelphia: Elsevier Saunders; 2010. p. 271–94.

14. Hobson SA, Karantana A, Dhar S. Total ankle replacement in patients with significant pre-operative deformity of the hindfoot. J Bone Joint Surg Br 2009;91:481–6.

15. Myerson MS. Revision total ankle replacement. Chapter 25. In: Myerson MS, editor. Reconstructive foot and ankle surgery: management of complications. 2nd edition. Philadelphia: Elsevier Saunders; 2010. p. 295–316.

16. Gupta S, Ellington JK, Myerson MS. Management of specific complications after revision total ankle replacement. Semin Arthroplasty 2010;21:310–9.

17. Jonck JH, Myerson MS. Revision total ankle replacement. Foot Ankle Clin 2012;7: 687–706.

18. McCollum G, Myerson MS. Failure of the Agility Total Ankle Replacement System and the salvage options. Clin Podiatr Med Surg 2013;30:207–23.

19. DeOrio JK, Lewis JS Jr. Silfverskiöld's test in total ankle replacement with gastrocnemius recession. Foot Ankle Int 2014;35:116–22.

20. Ketz J, Myerson M, Sanders R. The salvage of complex hindfoot problems with use of a custom talar total ankle prosthesis. J Bone Joint Surg Am 2012;94: 1194–200.

21. Queen RM, Grier AJ, Butler RJ, et al. The influence of concomitant triceps surae lengthening at the time of total ankle arthroplasty on postoperative outcomes. Foot Ankle Int 2014;35(9):863–70.

22. Gérard R, Unno-Veith F, Fasel J, et al. The effect of collateral ligament release on ankle dorsiflexion: an anatomical study. J Foot Ankle Surg 2011;17:193–6.

23. Schweinberger MH, Roukis TS. Surgical correction of soft-tissue ankle equinus contracture. Clin Podiatr Med Surg 2008;25:571–85.

The Salto Talaris XT Revision Ankle Prosthesis

Thomas S. Roukis, DPM, PhD

KEYWORDS

- Agility total ankle replacement system • INBONE total ankle replacement system
- Salto Talaris total ankle replacement system
- Scandinavian total ankle replacement system • Total ankle arthroplasty

KEY POINTS

- Revision of failed total ankle replacement systems available for use in the United States remains challenging with little published guidance available.
- Explantation of a failed total ankle replacement with conversion to an alternative total ankle replacement system represents a viable option but is associated with an unacceptably high incidence of complications.
- The Salto Talaris XT Revision Ankle Prosthesis was designed for primary and revision total ankle replacement and its design optimizes surface area, cortical contact, and ultra-high-molecular-weight polyethylene (UHMWPE) conformity. Developed specifically to revise failed Salto Talaris Anatomic Ankle Prosthesis, although it has some limitations, it appears well suited to revise each of the total ankle replacement systems available for use in the United States.
- Design features of the Salto Talaris XT Revision Ankle Prosthesis include 2 tibial designs (standard conical plug with central short keel and a long-stemmed version), a flat cut talar component that has additional height and a long central peg stabilized with a posterior blade as well as multiple thicker UHMWPE inserts.
- However, even thicker UHMPWE inserts, wider tibial base plates, longer stemmed talar components, and augmented height tibial and talar components are needed to expand the ability for the Salto Talaris XT Revision Ankle Prosthesis to be universally capable of reliably revising all failed total ankle replacement encountered in the United States.

INTRODUCTION

Total ankle replacement is a demanding procedure that can ultimately fail for myriad reasons and require revision. As proposed by Henricson and colleagues,[1] the specific definitions for secondary procedures performed for failed total ankle

Financial Disclosure: None reported.
Conflict of Interest: None reported.
Orthopaedic Center, Gundersen Health System, Mail Stop: CO2-006, 1900 South Avenue, La Crosse, WI 54601, USA
E-mail address: tsroukis@gundersenhealth.org

replacement include (1) revision, defined as any removal or exchange of one or more of the metallic prosthesis components except for incidental exchange of the ultra-high-molecular-weight polyethylene (UHMWPE) insert (ie, metallic component replacement, custom prosthesis utilization, ankle or tibiotalocalcaneal arthrodesis, or below-knee amputation); (2) reoperation, defined as nonrevisional secondary surgery involving the joint (ie, debridement, incidental UHMWPE insert exchange, or wound treatment); and (3) additional procedure, defined as nonrevisional secondary surgery not involving the joint (eg, ligament reconstruction/release, adjacent joint arthrodesis, adjacent periarticular osteotomy, or tendon lengthening/transfer).

The US public can receive only 1 of 9 metal-backed fixed-bearing cemented total ankle replacement devices that are 510(k) cleared and one 3-component, mobile-bearing, uncemented device conditionally approved by the US Food and Drug Administration (FDA) for general use. The metal-backed fixed-bearing cemented total ankle replacement devices that have been FDA cleared for use include the following:

- Agility and Agility LP Total Ankle Replacement Systems (DePuy Orthopedics, Inc, Warsaw, IN, USA)
- INBONE I, INBONE II, and INFINITY Total Ankle Replacement Systems (Wright Medical Technology, Inc, Arlington, TN, USA)
- Eclipse (Integra LifeSciences, Plainsboro, NJ, USA)
- Salto Talaris Anatomic Ankle Prosthesis and Salto Talaris XT Revision Ankle Prosthesis (Tornier, Inc, Bloomington, MN, USA/Wright Medical Technology, Inc)
- Zimmer Trabecular Metal Total Ankle (Zimmer, Inc, Warsaw, IN, USA)

In addition, one 3-component mobile-bearing uncemented total ankle replacement has received FDA premarket approval for use, the Scandinavian Total Ankle Replacement system (STAR; Stryker Orthopaedics, Inc, Mahwah, NJ, USA).

Based on the specific definitions for secondary procedures proposed by Henricson and colleagues,[1] the incidence of revision following primary implantation of the Agility Total Ankle Replacement System has been determined to be 10.2% (240 revisions/2353 primary implants) at a weighted mean follow-up of 24.1 months.[2,3] Specifically, 77.1% (185/240) of the revisions consisted of implant component replacement followed by ankle arthrodesis (44/240; 18.3% of revisions) and below-knee amputation (11/240; 4.6% of revisions).[2,3] Excluding the inventor increased the incidence nearly 2-fold, from 7.8% (84/1074) to 13% (172/1320), implicating potential selection (inventor) bias.[2,3] It should be noted that all studies included in this systematic review involved an uncemented Agility Total Ankle Replacement that is against the FDA requirements for the 510(k) cleared use of this prosthesis. Furthermore, the implant evaluated was the version available for use between 1998 and 2007, but the exact version of the talar component implanted (ie, original, posterior augmented, revision) could not be determined. Data pertaining to the Agility LP Total Ankle Replacement System, which became available for use in 2007, have not been published; however, an FDA clinical trial conducted by noninventor/paid consultants completed in November 2012 determined an incidence of revision of 6% (3/50) at a mean follow-up of 24 months (http://www.clinicaltrials.gov/ct2/show/results/NCT01366872?term=Agility+LP&rank=1&sect=X867015#outcome3; Last accessed: July 15, 2015). However, these investigators noted radiographic findings of talar subsidence at final follow-up in 10 (20%), both talar and tibial subsidence in 5 (10%), and tibial subsidence in 1 (2%). Because metallic component subsidence is a known potential precursor to revision,[2,4] the overall incidence of metallic component subsidence of 32% (16/50) is a cause for concern, and it would be beneficial for these investigators to publish their medium- and long-term follow-up of these patients.

Similarly, the incidence of revision following primary implantation of the STAR system has been determined to be 10.7% (269/2507) at a weighted mean follow-up of 64 months.[5] The specific revision performed was not clearly defined for 51.7% (139/269) prostheses. For the remaining prostheses, revision consisted of metallic component replacement 50.7% (66/130) followed by ankle arthrodesis (62/130; 47.7%) and below-knee/above-knee amputation (2/130; 1.5% of revisions). Excluding the inventor or paid faculty consultants increased the incidence more than 2-fold, from 5.6% (45/807) to 13.2% (224/1700), implicating potential selection (inventor) and publication (conflict of interest) bias.

The incidence of revision following primary implantation of the INBONE I Total Ankle Replacement system is elusive, but 2 articles include details of the incidence of complications leading to revision of 13.2% (7/53) at a weighted mean follow-up of 29.2 months.[6,7] All revisions were performed for talar component subsidence and the specific revision performed consisted of subtalar joint arthrodesis, 71.4% (5/7), with one of these included polymethylmethacrylate (PMMA) augmentation and talar component exchange and tibiotalocalcaneal arthrodesis, 14.3% (1/7). One patient requiring revision was lost to follow-up. It should be noted that both of these studies involved an uncemented INBONE I Total Ankle Replacement that is against the FDA requirements for the 510(k) cleared use of this prosthesis.

In contrast with the above, the Salto Talaris Total Ankle Prostheses was determined to have an incidence of revision of 2.1% (4 revisions/189 primary implants) at a weighted mean follow-up of 34.8 months.[8] Specifically, 3 metallic component replacements and one ankle arthrodesis were performed. Restricting the data to the inventor, design team, or disclosed consultants, the incidence of revision was 2.6% and, in contrast, data that excluded these individuals had an incidence of revision of 1.3% for the Salto Talaris Total Ankle Prostheses.

The remaining metal-backed fixed-bearing cemented total ankle replacement devices that have been FDA 510(k) cleared for use have no published clinical data such that determination of the incidence of complications requiring revision remains unknown.

Revision of failed total ankle replacement remains a vexing problem with limited proven approaches. In the United States, revision of the failed STAR system is limited to thicker UHMWPE inserts and potentially explantation with conversion to the INBONE II Total Ankle Replacement System, Salto Talaris Total Ankle Prosthesis, or Salto Talaris XT Revision Ankle Prosthesis (**Figs. 1–4**). Unfortunately, no published articles detail the use of these prostheses following explantation of the failed STAR system. As described for the Agility Total Ankle Replacement System, when feasible, isolated talar component and UHMWPE revision represent a low risk and fiscally sound option.[9,10] One alternative component revision strategy is custom-designed long-stemmed tibial or talar components[10–15] that allow augmentation of segmental bone loss and spanning fixation into the tibial metaphysis or calcaneus. Another is explantation and conversion to an alternative total ankle replacement system available for use in the United States, specifically, the INBONE II Total Ankle Replacement System[10,16–19] and Salto Talaris Total Ankle Prosthesis[20,21] or Salto Talaris XT Revision Ankle Prosthesis[10,20] (**Figs. 5 and 6**). Revision INBONE I Total Ankle Replacement with the talar component supported by metal-reinforced triangular

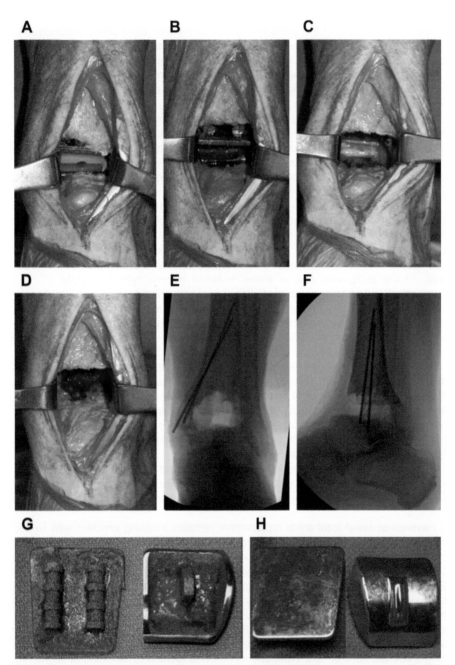

Fig. 1. Intraoperative photograph demonstrating a failed STAR (*A*). Following removal of the UHMWPE insert, the tibial and talar components are gently pried from the underlying bone in that order (*B*) and removed (*C*). Intraoperative photograph demonstrating well-vascularized residual talar body despite medial and posterior talar bone loss (*D*). Image intensification mortise (*E*) and lateral (*F*) ankle radiographs demonstrating the residual osseous defect. Note the retained internal fixation used to fixate an intraoperative medial malleolar fracture during the index surgery. Intraoperative photograph of the failed STAR demonstrating lack of osseous ongrowth (*G*) and extensive abrasion of the tibial and talar surfaces (*H*).

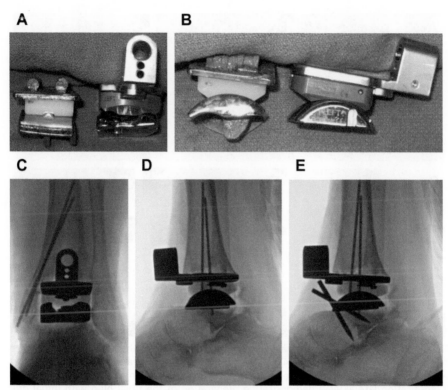

Fig. 2. Intraoperative photograph demonstrating anterior (*A*) and lateral (*B*) views of the failed STAR relative to the Salto Talaris XT Revision Ankle Prosthesis trial components. Image intensification mortise (*C*) and lateral (*D*) views following insertion of the Salto Talaris XT Revision Ankle Prosthesis trial components and completion of "dynamic flexion and extension range of motion" demonstrating optimal component alignment. Image intensification lateral view demonstrating pin insertion through the talar trial component and into the talar body without violating the subtalar joint (*E*).

rods/large-diameter screws affixed within a PMMA cement mantle,[22] permanent PMMA cement spacer,[23–25] TTC arthrodesis with bulk intercalary allograft,[26–28] or below-knee amputation[26] should be reserved for select non-reconstructable cases, uncontrollable deep periprosthetic infection, or situations where the patient does not desire or is medically unable to undergo revision surgery.

Unfortunately, as of December 8, 2011, any custom-design long-stemmed talar component is no longer available for clinical use in the United States because of FDA regulation, and the availability of this in the future remains uncertain (http://www.fda.gov/ICECI/EnforcementActions/WarningLetters/2011/ucm287552.htm; Last accessed: July 15, 2015). Alternatively, explantation with conversion to the INBONE I or INBONE II Total Ankle Replacement system as a "megaprosthesis" is warranted when other options are not feasible and the osseous defect is massive such that even TTC with bulk intercalary allograft would be challenging. However, this is time-consuming, fraught with potential catastrophic complications, and is considered a limb-salvage procedure.[16–19] DeVries and colleagues[16] reported an incidence of complications of 64.3% (9/14) with Agility Total Ankle Replacement explantation and conversion to the INBONE I Total Ankle Replacement. Meeker and colleagues[17] reported

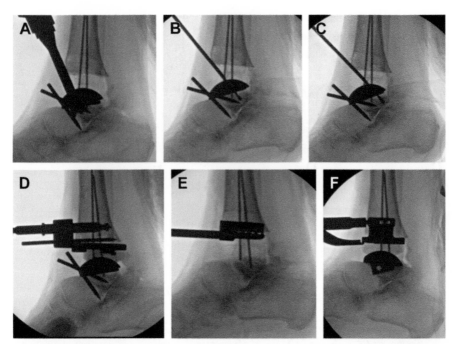

Fig. 3. Image intensification lateral views demonstrating use of the bell-shaped reamer to create the hole for the talar peg (*A*) followed by drilling the more anterior (*B*) and then posterior (*C*) of the holes used to create the posterior blade portion of the talar peg. Image intensification lateral view demonstrating preparation of the tibial plug with initial drill bit advancement through the most proximal hole (*D*) followed by keel preparation with a dedicated bone impaction rasp (*E*). Image intensification lateral view demonstrating insertion of the tibial assembly (*F*) that follows insertion of the talar component.

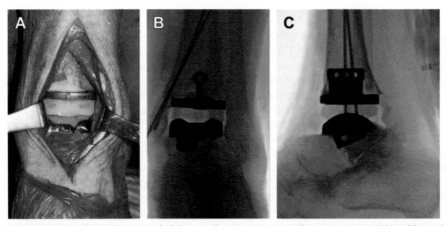

Fig. 4. Intraoperative photograph (*A*) as well as image intensification mortise (*B*) and lateral (*C*) ankle views following explantation of the failed STAR and conversion to a Salto Talaris XT Revision Ankle Prosthesis. Note the impaction grafting of cancellous bone into the talar defect and PMMA cement about the anterior tibial cortical defect and prosthesis keel/plug.

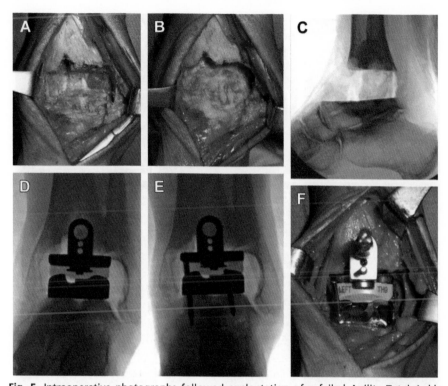

Fig. 5. Intraoperative photographs followed explantation of a failed Agility Total Ankle Replacement system demonstrating the extensive osseous defect (*A*) and sclerotic talar body about the talar keel channel (*B*). Image intensification lateral view demonstrating the resultant flat tibial and talar surfaces obtained following use of a small power saw and hand rasps (*C*). Intraoperative image intensification mortise ankle view following insertion of the Salto Talaris XT Revision Ankle Prosthesis tibial assembly and talar trial components demonstrating proper component alignment (*D*). Intraoperative image intensification mortise ankle following pinning of the talar component (*E*). Intraoperative photograph demonstrating fixation of the tibial trial component with a distal pin and proximal drill and talar component with 2 offset pins (*F*). Note that despite the massive osseous defect created following removal of the failed Agility Total Ankle Replacement, it was not necessary to use a thicker revision poly to achieve proper ligamentous tension. In this case, a 6-mm poly trial is used, which when combined with the 3-mm-thick tibial trial results in a 9-mm-thick tibial assembly (Th 9 noted on the yellow trial poly).

an incidence of complications of 27.7% (5/18) with Agility Total Ankle Replacement explantation and conversion to the INBONE II Total Ankle Replacement. Williams and colleagues[19] from the same institution as Meeker and colleagues[17] reported an overall incidence of complications of 31.4% (11/35) with Agility Total Ankle Replacement explantation and conversion to the INBONE II Total Ankle Replacement. Finally, Roukis and Simonson,[10] detailing their learning curve experience with revision total ankle replacement, reported an incidence of complications of 75% (6/8) with Agility Total Ankle Replacement explantation and conversion to the INBONE II Total Ankle Replacement. In summary, the overall incidence of complications with Agility Total Ankle Replacement explantation and conversion to the INBONE I or INBONE II Total Ankle Replacement was 41.3%.[10,16,17,19] Although it is obviously beneficial to have

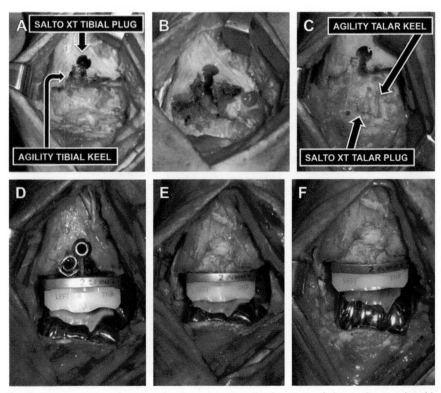

Fig. 6. Intraoperative photographs demonstrating the location of the Agility Total Ankle Replacement tibial keel relative to the Salto Talaris XT Revision Ankle Prosthesis tibial keel and plug (*A*). The extensive loss of cancellous bone within the tibial plafond medially and sclerotic bone mantle laterally is demonstrated (*B*). Intraoperative photograph demonstrating the location of the Agility Total Ankle Replacement talar keel relative to the Salto Talaris XT Revision Ankle Prosthesis talar plug (*C*). Intraoperative photograph following implantation of the final Salto Talaris XT Revision Ankle Prosthesis demonstrating metal reinforcement within the medial distal tibial osseous defect adjacent to the keel of the tibial component (*D*) followed by PMMA cement augmentation (*E*). Intraoperative photograph demonstrating complete talar body coverage but only partial tibial coverage due to the specific dimensions of the osseous defect created by explantation of the Agility Total Ankle Replacement system (*F*). Note the very thin residual medial malleolus.

a total ankle replacement system capable of revising the massive osseous defects created with explantation of the Agility Total Ankle Replacement system, the incidence of complications using the INBONE I or INBONE II Total Ankle Replacement systems is unacceptable. The Salto Talaris XT Revision Ankle Prosthesis was developed to specifically revise failed Salto Talaris Anatomic Ankle Prosthesis but seems ideally suited to revise each of the total ankle replacement systems available for use in the United States.

SALTO TALARIS XT REVISION ANKLE PROSTHESIS

The Salto Talaris XT Revision Ankle Prosthesis (**Fig. 7**) is indicated for primary and revision total ankle replacement and has been cleared by the FDA only for use with PMMA

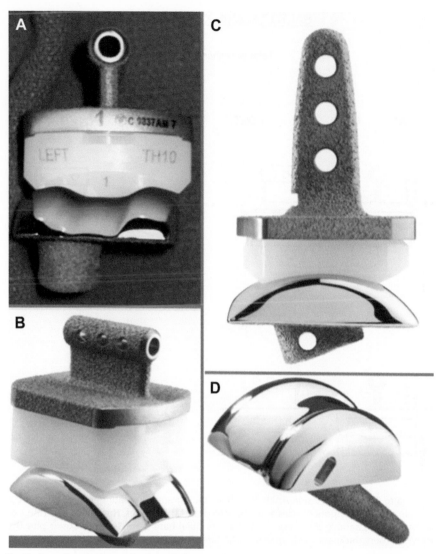

Fig. 7. Anterior photograph of the fully assembled Salto Talaris XT Revision Ankle Prosthesis (*A*). Photograph of the standard tibial component affixed to a thicker revision UHMWPE insert and XT revision talar component (*B*). Lateral photograph of the long-stemmed tibial component affixed to a standard UHMWPE insert and XT revision talar component (*C*). Photograph of the long-stemmed XT revision talar component (*D*).

cement fixation. The Salto Talaris XT Revision Ankle Prosthesis consists of size 1, 2, and 3 tibial and talar components (**Fig. 8**) and is based off of the Salto Talaris Anatomic Ankle Prosthesis design. No size 0 is available for the Salto Talaris XT Revision Ankle Prosthesis. Both the tibial and the talar components are made of cobalt-chromium and are single-coated with 200-μm plasma-sprayed titanium (T40) to promote osseous integration. The standard tibial base plate is identical between systems, and component fixation is achieved primarily with anterior cortical contact of the flat surface and a 12-mm-long central keel attached to a hollow tapered anterior-posterior conical

SALTO TALARIS XT - Standard associations

Talar part short peg - Right model

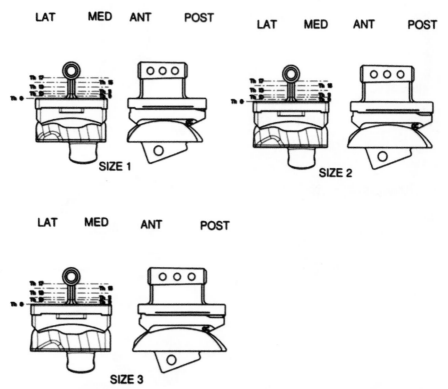

Fig. 8. Salto Talaris XT Revision Ankle Prosthesis radiograph template demonstrating the 3 available metallic component sizes and UHMWPE insert thicknesses. Note that "Th" refers to the total tibial assembly thickness defined as the tibial base plate 3-mm-thickness plus the UHMWPE insert thickness. ANT, anterior; LAT, lateral; MED, medial; POST, posterior.

fixation plug that is impacted into the tibial metaphysis. The standard tibial component is designed for insertion with 7° or 3° posterior slope relative to the long-axis of the tibia. A stemmed tibial component with a 40-mm-long central keel (see **Fig. 7**C) will soon be released for general use in the United States but has been available by surgeon prescription only on a compassionate use basis since 2012. The tibial base can be the same or one size larger than the talar component, allowing for mismatching the tibial and talar components based on patient anatomy. The tibial components are interchangeable, but the talar components have dedicated left and right sides due to the double radii (ie, medial radius smaller than lateral radius) and biconvex articular surface resembling the native morphology of the talar dome. The talar component has deep biconvex medial and lateral articular surfaces with a concave trochlear groove and a 12° apex medial frontal plane axis to allow for external rotation of the foot with dorsiflexion and internal rotation during plantarflexion. The anatomic design of the talar component is intended to reproduce normal ankle kinematics without overstressing the deltoid ligament complex. Compared with the Salto Talaris Anatomic Ankle Prosthesis talar height of 5.5 mm, the Salto Talaris XT Revision Prosthesis talar component has greater height, being 10.5 mm for size 1, 11.4 mm for size 2, and 11.9 mm for size 3. The undersurface of the talar component is flat, and primary stability involves a 70°posterior angled 10.2-mm-deep 12-mm outer diameter medially offset hollow fixation peg with a stabilizing posterior blade. Additional flat-cut talar long 55-mm stemmed components (see **Fig. 7**D) are pending release for use in the United States, one with 2-mm greater height and the other with 9-mm posterior augmentation. The UHMWPE inserts are available in the standard thicknesses of 5, 6, 7, and 8 mm and revision thicknesses of 10, 12, and 14 mm (see **Fig. 7**B) with 16- and 18-mm thicknesses planned for eventual release. (Note: These measures are the actual thicknesses, not the composite thicknesses used to describe the tibial assembly consisting of the tibial component base plate thickness of 3 mm plus the actual UHMWPE thickness.) The UHMWPE inserts articular surface is size matched to the talar component and have dedicated left and right sides. The contact area between the UHMWPE insert and talar component allows ±2-mm varus/valgus motion, 5° internal/external rotation, 2-mm anterior-to-posterior translation, and a sagittal plane arc of motion from 20° dorsiflexion and 25° plantarflexion.

SURGICAL APPROACH

During revision of all total ankle replacement systems available for use in the United States, a standard anterior ankle incision is used, taking care to protect the anterior neurovascular bundle and maintain appropriate tissue planes for layered closure, while minimizing retraction to only what is necessary to preserve the tenuous anterior soft tissues.[29] It should be noted that any retained deep metallic hardware that would interfere with placement of the Salto Talaris XT Revision Ankle Prosthesis is removed first unless it would best be accomplished through the anterior ankle incision. After entry into the ankle joint space, the periosteal tissues are elevated directly off the bone overlying the tibial component and then the talar component. Soft tissue exposure is limited to only what is needed to visualize the metallic components along with the medial and lateral gutters (see **Fig. 1**A). Once soft tissue dissection is completed, the UHMWPE insert is removed (see **Fig. 1**B).

For the Agility Total Ankle Replacement system, the talar component is freed from ectopic bone growth and then gently pried free of the underlying bone with care taken not to fracture the talus during manipulation. Removal of the tibial component follows and most commonly involves first curetting any osteolysis regions about the perimeter and then separating the interface between the prosthesis porous coating and native bone. Remarkably sound osseous ongrowth to the tibial component is commonly encountered. Therefore, this step needs to be performed very carefully to avoid cutting through the malleoli with the saw excursion or fracturing the distal tibia with incomplete separation of the prosthesis and bone during attempted mobilization of the tibial component. It is intuitive that these same steps would be used for removal of the failed Salto Talaris Total Ankle Prosthesis as well as the INBONE I, INBONE II, and INFINITY Total Ankle Replacement systems. However, for the failed STAR system, the tibial component needs to be removed first to create enough space to remove the talar component. The Zimmer Trabecular Metal Total Ankle would need to be cut out with flat cuts because of the curved design, intense Trabecular metal bonding to the adjacent bone, and use of PMMA adjacent to the metallic component rails.

TIBIAL AND TALAR RESECTION

The accuracy of tibial component alignment using the Salto Talaris Anatomic Ankle Prosthesis, which is the same as the Salto Talaris XT Revision Ankle Prosthesis, extramedullary referencing guide was tested in 83 ankles and determined to be within a mean of 1.5° and 4.1° in the coronal and sagittal planes, respectively, from the surgeons intended position.[30] However, because explantation of the failed total ankle replacement tibial component most commonly results in a flat distal tibial plafond and vertical gutter surfaces, the use of the tibial alignment guide routinely proves unnecessary. Any uneven surfaces are smoothed with a combination of a small power saw and various sized hand rasps and cystic regions curetted until bleeding cancellous substrate is exposed (see **Fig. 1**D). Occasionally, the most medial and lateral aspects of the distal tibia are extremely sclerotic, such that resection of nearly the entire distal tibial plafond would be required to expose viable bone. In these situations, it is advantageous to retain the sclerotic bone for structural support and perform multiple fenestrations to expose subchondral bone with the intention of either "spot weld bonding" with the tibial component or to increase the contact area of the PMMA cement within the bone (see **Fig. 6**B). Care should be taken to verify that the distal end of the tibial plafond is parallel with the floor or perpendicular to the mechanical axis of the tibia. The medial and lateral gutters adjacent to the talar body and malleoli are resected of soft tissue and bone debris to reduce impingement and improve sagittal plane range of motion. Next, the talar body is converted to a flat surface free of frontal or sagittal plane biased resection. This conversion is most commonly performed with a combination of a small power saw and various sized hand rasps. The previous total ankle replacements talar fixation keel region is usually very sclerotic, and care should be taken to remove this sclerotic bone and expose cancellous substrate (see **Fig. 6**C). If the defect is substantial, then cancellous impaction bone grafting in young patients with a well-vascularized talus or metal-reinforced PMMA filling in older patients with osteoporotic bone is performed.

TRIAL SIZE EVALUATION AND IMPLANT SELECTION

The trial components are assembled based on the measured osseous defect with the foot held in slight distraction at the ankle joint to tension the medial and lateral ligaments. For the standard and revision UHMWPE, the tibial trial base and poly trial insert are clipped together and the selected talar trial implant is then implanted as a unit (see **Fig. 5**F). Comparing the various combinations of components to the explanted failed total ankle replacement facilitates the assembly of the Salto Talaris XT Revision Ankle Prosthesis trial components (see **Fig. 2**A, B). The trial components are initially inserted into the osseous defect with the foot in slight plantarflexion. An assistant then applies direct linear distal traction on the foot while the surgeon manually impacts the components into the osseous defect. Next, the trial components are allowed to rotate into proper position during sagittal ankle range of motion termed "dynamic flexion and extension range of motion test" in the technique guide. Care is taken to make certain that there is symmetric tension on the medial and lateral ligament complexes (see **Fig. 2**C) and that the tibial and talar trial components are properly aligned (see **Fig. 2**D) before pinning the construct to bone (see **Fig. 2**E). This alignment is best accomplished by first verifying direct contact between the laser line etching on the anterior aspect of the tibial trial base and the anterior tibia. Next, it is important to ensure that the talar trial has maximum talar body coverage and is not anteriorly or posteriorly translated relative to the lateral process of the talus that should be under the center of the component. Furthermore, it is imperative to confirm that the entire construct is rotationally aligned with the second metatarsal and not excessively internally or externally rotated. The final step involves performing stress inversion and eversion to check the lateral and medial ligament complex stability, respectively. These steps are critical and should be repeatedly checked and verified as accurate before and after pinning the talar trial into place using two 45-mm pins. The medial pin is more vertically oriented than the lateral pin that is more horizontal (see **Figs. 2**E and **5**D). Applying a light coat of mineral oil to the pins and initially aligning them manually help to ease insertion. The tibial trial base and trial poly insert are removed and the hole for the talar peg is drilled through the corresponding hole in the talar trial using the bell-shaped reamer (see **Fig. 3**A) provided in the Salto Talaris XT Revision Ankle prosthesis instrumentation not the one in the Salto Talaris Anatomic Ankle Prosthesis. It is important to avoid direct contact between the hard stop flange on the reamer and the talar trial because this will cause the metallic parts to bind. If binding occurs, rotation of the talar trial can cause catastrophic problems, including fracture of the talar neck about the pin sites and malleolar fractures. Instead, the reamer is advanced until it nearly contacts the talar trial and is then withdrawn without stopping. The resultant partial talar hole for the talar peg is completed after removing the talar trial but before tibial preparation. Next, the talar flange position posterior to the talar peg is predrilled through 2 drill holes in the talar trial (see **Fig. 3**B, C). The pins and talar trial are removed and the hole for the talar peg is further reamed to complete the preparation followed by completing the slot for the posterior blade portion of the talar peg using the tibial flange osteotome and a small angled curette. It is important not to penetrate the inferior aspect of the talar body with any of the pins or drills in order to prevent damage to the artery of the tarsal canal.[31] It is intuitive that proper metallic pin and drill insertion technique and liberal use of intraoperative C-arm image intensification will reduce this risk pattern. The talar trial is reinserted and the talar fixation plug is placed through the talar trial to fix the components position. With the talar component preparation finalized, the tibial trial with poly insert previously chosen are reinserted to determine the final tibial component positioning using the dynamic flexion and extension range of motion test. Once the tibial base plate is verified as resting in the optimum position, the tibial keel is prepared. The inferior 2 holes are drilled and a 45-mm pin in the distal hole is left to hold the trial tibial base in place, followed by preparation of the tibial plug with a drill bit through the trial's most proximal hole (see **Fig. 3**D). Because the tibial component position is usually more proximal in the tibia during revision total ankle replacement compared with primary cases, care must be taken not to inadvertently drill through the posterior tibial cortex because this can lead to fracture of the tibia. The trial tibial base and poly insert are removed, and the keel is completed with the tibial flange osteotome and bone impaction rasp (see **Fig. 3**E) with care taken not to inadvertently fracture the anterior tibial cortex, especially in cases where the Agility Total Ankle Replacement is being revised because the tibial keel for this system is directly adjacent to the standard and stemmed Salto Talaris XT Revision Ankle Prosthesis tibial keel (see **Fig. 6**A). For the stemmed tibial component, the anterior tibial cortex is windowed to allow for room to insert the tibial keel followed by levering into the intramedullary tibial canal. Care must be taken not to lever off and inadvertently fracture the posterior tibia nor rotate the component and fracture the malleoli. Alternatively, the tibial component preparation can be completed before the talar component; this is useful in situations where is it difficult to capture proper component rotation while maintaining anterior tibial cortical coverage of the tibial trial component.

Following copious irrigation, the surgical site cystic lesions within the tibia or talus are impaction grafted with cancellous bone in younger patients who have broad exposure of native cancellous bone substrate complemented by a thin layer of antibiotic impregnated PMMA cement (Simplex P with Tobramycin; Stryker Orthopaedics) about the perimeter of the replaced metallic components to provide immediate stability. The talar component is inserted first and impacted into the talus followed by impaction of the tibial assembly (ie, tibial component with affixed UHMWPE insert). In situations involving advanced osteolysis and resultant contained osseous defects from cyst formation, especially in elderly patients with associated osteopenia, metal-reinforced antibiotic impregnated PMMA cement is used to back-fill the osseous defect and secondarily provide some stability to the metallic components (see **Fig. 6**D, E).[18,32–34]

POSTOPERATIVE CARE

Meticulous, layered closure is essential. Every patient receives a surgical drain and an anterior windowed folded Webril Undercast Padding (Kendall-Coviden, Mansfield, MA, USA) cutout to the anterior incision line to limit pressure on the anterior incision line.[10] This is followed by a Sir Robert Jones compression dressing and posterior molded plaster splint for edema reduction during the postoperative period.[35] All patients follow the author's standard postoperative protocol for total ankle replacement as previously described.[31,36] At the 8-week follow-up appointment, weight-bearing ankle radiographs are obtained and, if no complications are noted, patients are permitted to transition into full weight-bearing and back into a supportive shoe or lace-up high-topped boot. Weight-bearing ankle radiographs are obtained including stress sagittal plane dorsiflexion and plantarflexion as well as long leg axial[37] views 1 year from the revision total ankle replacement and every year thereafter during the annual surveillance program used by the author. Although controversial, dental antibiotic prophylaxis, use of a brace or lace-up high-topped boot with any exposure to uneven ground, and avoidance of ballistic activities is enforced lifelong.

COMPLICATIONS

Explantation of failed total ankle replacement systems with conversion to alternative total ankle replacement systems is associated with myriad intraoperative and perioperative complications that can negatively affect outcome. Therefore, the surgeon and patient should expect a high incidence of complications to occur with revision total ankle replacement performed through explantation and conversion of systems. Specific to the Salto Talaris XT Revision Ankle Prosthesis, explantation and conversion are viable options when limited bone loss exists. However, until thicker UHMPWE inserts, wider tibial base plates, long-stemmed talar, and augmented height tibial and talar components are readily available, it remains underpowered for universal revision of failed total ankle replacements especially the Agility and Agility LP Total Ankle Replacement systems as well as the INBONE I and INBONE II Total Ankle Replacement systems.

Another concern involves the complexity involved in properly seating the long-stemmed tibial component as well as unequal dispersion of load about the subarticular bone adjacent to the standard tibial keel and conical fixation plug especially with limited prosthesis to viable native bone contact. Specifically, the location of osteolysis concentrated around the standard tibial keel and conical fixation plug for the Salto Mobile Version prosthesis (Tornier NV, Amsterdam, The Netherlands) correlates exactly with increased load transmission and strain during thermoelastic stress analysis[38] and finite element modeling.[39] Therefore, further refinement of the tibial component to ease insertion of the long-stemmed version as well as redistribute stress for more even dispersion of load should be areas of future study. Access to the HINTEGRA Ankle Prosthesis (Newdeal, Lyon, France/Integra) that has established revision total ankle prosthesis components available for use outside the United States capable of revising failed STAR systems[40,41] would be meaningful. Clearly, there is a real need for outcome studies to evaluate patients undergoing revision total ankle replacement for the current prosthesis systems available in the United States and abroad, and future efforts ought to be directed in this area.

SUMMARY

Explantation of a failed total ankle replacement with conversion to the Salto Talaris XT Revision Ankle Prosthesis seems to be a viable option when limited bone loss exists, especially about the distal tibial metaphysis. Following explantation of the failed total ankle replacement, implantation of the Salto Talaris XT Revision Ankle Prosthesis involves only a few straightforward steps for accurate implantation. The ability to mismatch the tibial and talar components one size is beneficial when the tibial defect is wider than the available talar surface such as when revising failed Agility Total Ankle Replacements. However, until thicker UHMPWE inserts, wider tibial base plates, long-stemmed talar components, and augmented height tibial and talar components are readily available, it remains underpowered for universal use with revision of failed total ankle replacement systems available for use in the United States.

REFERENCES

1. Henricson A, Carlsson Å, Rydholm U. What is a revision of total ankle replacement? Foot Ankle Surg 2011;17:99–102.
2. Roukis TS. Incidence of revision after primary implantation of the Agility total ankle replacement system: a systematic review. J Foot Ankle Surg 2012;51: 198–204.
3. Criswell BJ, Douglas K, Naik R. High revision and reoperation rates using the Agility Total Ankle System. Clin Orthop Relat Res 2012;(470):1980–6.
4. Lee AY, Ha AS, Petscavage JM, et al. Total ankle arthroplasty: a radiographic outcome study. AJR Am J Roentgenol 2013;200:1310–6.
5. Prissel MA, Roukis TS. Incidence of revision after primary implantation of the Scandinavian total ankle replacement system: a systematic review. Clin Podiatr Med Surg 2013;30:237–50.
6. Datir A, Xing M, Kakarala A, et al. Radiographic evaluation of INBONE total ankle arthroplasty: a retrospective analysis of 30 cases. Skeletal Radiol 2013;42: 1693–701.
7. Brigido SA, Galli MM, Bleazey ST, et al. Modular stem-fixed bearing total ankle replacement: prospective results of 23 consecutive cases with 3-year follow-up. J Foot Ankle Surg 2014;53:692–9.
8. Roukis TS, Elliot AD. Incidence of revision following primary implantation of the Salto Mobile Version and Salto Talaris Total Ankle Prostheses: a systematic review. J Foot Ankle Surg 2015;54:311–9.

9. Gould JS. Revision total ankle arthroplasty. Am J Orthop 2005;34:361.

10. Roukis TS, Simonson DC. Incidence of complications during initial experience with revision of the Agility and Agility LP total ankle replacement systems: a single surgeon's learning curve experience. Clin Podiatr Med Surg 2015, in press.

11. Ellington JK, Gupta S, Myerson MS. Management of failures of total ankle replacement with the agility total ankle arthroplasty. J Bone Joint Surg Am 2013;95-A:2112–8.

12. Myerson MS, Won HY. Primary and revision total ankle replacement using custom-designed prosthesis. Foot Ankle Clin 2008;13:521–38.

13. Ketz J, Myerson M, Sanders R. The salvage of complex hindfoot problems with use of a custom talar total ankle prosthesis. J Bone Joint Surg Am 2012;94-A: 1194–200.

14. Noriega F, Villanueva P, Moracia I, et al. Custom-made talar component in primary young patients and total ankle replacement revision: short-term results. J Bone Joint Surg Am 2011;93-B(Suppl. II):148.

15. Roukis TS. Salvage of a failed DePuy Alvine Total Ankle Prosthesis with Agility LP custom stemmed tibia and talar components. Clin Podiatr Med Surg 2013;30: 101–9.

16. DeVries JG, Scott RT, Berlet GC, et al. Agility to INBONE: anterior and posterior approaches to the difficult revision total ankle replacement. Clin Podiatr Med Surg 2013;30:81–96.

17. Meeker J, Wegner N, Francisco R, et al. Revision techniques in total ankle arthroplasty using a stemmed tibial arthroplasty system. Tech Foot Ankle Surg 2013;12: 99–108.

18. Roukis TS. Management of the failed Agility total ankle replacement system. Foot Ankle Quarterly 2013;24:185–97.

19. Williams JR, Wegner NJ, Sangeorzan BJ, et al. Intra-operative and peri-operative complications during revision arthroplasty for salvage of a failed total ankle arthroplasty. Foot Ankle Int 2015;36:135–42.

20. Jonck JH, Myerson MS. Revision total ankle replacement. Foot Ankle Clin N Am 2012;17:687–706.

21. McCollum G, Myerson MS. Failure of the Agility total ankle replacement system and salvage options. Clin Podiatr Med Surg 2013;30:207–23.

22. Schuberth JM, Christensen JC, Rialson JA. Metal-reinforced cement augmentation for complex talar subsidence in failed total ankle arthroplasty. J Foot Ankle Surg 2011;50:766–72.

23. Ferrao P, Myerson MS, Schuberth JM, et al. Cement spacer as definitive management for postoperative ankle infection. Foot Ankle Int 2012;33:173–8.

24. Myerson MS, Shariff R, Zonno AJ. The management of infection following total ankle replacement: demographics and treatment. Foot Ankle Int 2014;35: 855–62.

25. Lee H-S, Ahn J-Y, Lee J-S, et al. Cement arthroplasty for ankle joint destruction. J Bone Joint Surg Am 2014;96:1468–75.

26. Penner MJ. Failed ankle replacement and conversion to arthrodesis: a treatment algorithm. Tech Foot Ankle Surg 2012;11:125–32.

27. Donnenwerth M, Roukis TS. Tibio-talo-calcaneal arthrodesis with retrograde intramedullary compression nail fixation for salvage of failed total ankle replacement: a systematic review. Clin Podiatr Med Surg 2013;30:199–206.

28. DeOrio JK. Revision INBONE total ankle replacement. Clin Podiatr Med Surg 2013;30:225–36.

29. Raikin SM. Avoiding wound complications in total ankle arthroplasty: surgical technique and tips. J Bone Joint Surg Essential Surgical Techniques 2011;1-A: e6–11.
30. Adams SB Jr, Demetracopoulos CA, Viens NA, et al. Comparison of extramedullary versus intramedullary referencing for tibial component alignment in total ankle arthroplasty. Foot Ankle Int 2013;34:1624–8.
31. Schweinberger MH, Roukis TS. Effectiveness of instituting a specific bed protocol n reducing complications associated with bed rest. J Foot Ankle Surg 2010;49: 340–7.
32. Roukis TS, Prissel MA. Management of extensive tibial osteolysis with the Agility total ankle replacement systems using geometric metal-reinforced polymethylmethacrylate cement augmentation. J Foot Ankle Surg 2014;53:101–7.
33. Roukis TS, Prissel MA. Management of extensive talar osteolysis with the Agility total ankle replacement systems using geometric metal-reinforced polymethylmethacrylate cement augmentation. J Foot Ankle Surg 2014;53:108–13.
34. Roukis TS, Prissel MA. Revision of agility total ankle replacements using Agility components is the right choice, sometimes. J Foot Ankle Surg 2014;53:391–3.
35. Schade VL, Roukis TS. Use of a surgical preparation and sterile dressing change during office visit treatment of chronic foot and ankle wounds decreases the incidence of infection and treatment costs. Foot Ankle Spec 2008;1:147–54.
36. Abicht BP, Roukis TS. The INBONE II total ankle replacement system. Clin Podiatr Med Surg 2013;30:47–68.
37. Reilingh ML, Beimers L, Tuijthof GJ, et al. Measuring hindfoot alignment radiographically: the long axial view is more reliable than the hindfoot alignment view. Skeletal Radiol 2010;39:1103–8.
38. Ficklscherer A, Wegener B, Niethammer T, et al. Thermoelastic stress analysis to validate tibial fixation technique in total ankle prostheses: a pilot study. Ulus Travma Acil Cerrahi Derg 2013;19:98–102.
39. Terrier A, Larrea X, Guerdat J, et al. Development and experimental validation of a finite element model of total ankle replacement. J Biomech 2014;47:742–5.
40. Hintermann B, Zwicky L, Knupp M, et al. HINTEGRA revision arthroplasty for failed total ankle prostheses. J Bone Joint Surg Am 2013;95:1166–74.
41. Brunner S, Barg A, Knupp M, et al. The Scandinavian Total Ankle Replacement: long-term, eleven to fifteen-year, survivorship analysis of the prosthesis in seventy-two consecutive patients. J Bone Joint Surg Am 2013;95:711–8.

Incidence of Complications During Initial Experience with Revision of the Agility and Agility LP Total Ankle Replacement Systems

A Single Surgeon's Learning Curve Experience

Thomas S. Roukis, DPM, PhD*, Devin C. Simonson, DPM

KEYWORDS

- Complications • INBONE Total Ankle Replacement System
- Salto Talaris Total Ankle Replacement System • Salvage • Total ankle arthroplasty

KEY POINTS

- The Agility and Agility LP Total Ankle Replacement Systems were the primary prosthesis systems available for use in the United States for more than a decade, spanning 1998 to 2010.
- Surgeons unfamiliar with the primary implantation of the Agility and Agility LP Total Ankle Replacement Systems will likely encounter patients with failure of these prostheses that require revision. Revision of the failed Agility and Agility LP Total Ankle Replacement Systems is challenging with little published guidance available.
- Exchange of the Agility and Agility LP Total Ankle Replacement System components to Revision or LP talar components and ultrahigh-molecular-weight polyethylene (UHMWPE) insert with, in select instances, additional metal-reinforced polymethylmethacrylate cement augmentation; conversion to custom-designed stemmed components; or explantation and conversion to another total ankle replacement system are considerations.
- Custom-designed stemmed Agility LP Total Ankle Replacement is unfortunately no longer available because of US Food and Drug Administration regulation. Explantation with conversion to alternative total ankle replacement systems is a high-risk surgery with strong potential for complications to occur.
- Whenever feasible, exchange with Revision or LP talar components and UHMWPE insert with, in select instances, additional metal-reinforced polymethylmethacrylate cement augmentation remains a simple, low-cost, and viable option with limited occurrence of complications.

Financial Disclosure: None reported.

Conflict of Interest: None reported.

Orthopaedic Center, Gundersen Health System, Mail Stop: CO2-006, 1900 South Avenue, La Crosse, WI 54601, USA

* Corresponding author.

E-mail address: tsroukis@gundersenhealth.org

INTRODUCTION

Despite early generation failures, total ankle replacement (TAR) is now an established alternative to ankle arthrodesis for the treatment of end-stage ankle arthritis.[1–8] With the advent of third-generation TAR systems, foot and ankle surgeons competent in primary TAR have achieved clinical outcomes comparable to if not superior to ankle arthrodesis.[1–13] As the frequency in which foot and ankle surgeons are performing primary TAR continues to build, revision TAR will likely become more commonplace. This pattern has in fact been clearly demonstrated over time in the Norwegian Arthroplasty Register (http://nrlweb.ihelse.net/Rapporter/Rapport2014.pdf; Accessed July 18, 2015). Accordingly, there will be a need for an established benchmark by which to evaluate the safety of revision TAR as determined by the incidence of complications encountered. It seems intuitive that most complications occurring during primary TAR that lead to revision will occur during the surgeons' learning curve period. Although many reports exist suggesting the presence of a learning curve, there has been no large-scale published analysis of the exact incidence of complications encountered during the surgeon learning curve period for the primary TAR prosthesis systems available for current use.

At present, the US public can receive only 1 of 9 metal-backed fixed-bearing cemented TAR devices that are 510(k) cleared and one 3-component mobile-bearing uncemented device approved by the US Food and Drug Administration (FDA) for general use. The 9 metal-backed fixed-bearing cemented TAR devices that have been FDA cleared for use are (1) Agility and Agility LP Total Ankle Replacement Systems (DePuy Synthes Joint Reconstruction, Warsaw, IN, USA); (2) INBONE I, INBONE II, and INFINITY Total Ankle Replacement Systems (Wright Medical Technology, Inc, Arlington, TN, USA); (3) Eclipse (Integra LifeSciences, Plainsboro, NJ, USA); (4) Salto Talaris Anatomic Ankle Prosthesis and Salto Talaris XT Revision Ankle Prosthesis (Tornier, Bloomington, MN, USA); and (5) Zimmer Trabecular Metal Total Ankle (Zimmer, Inc, Warsaw, IN, USA). In addition, one 3-component mobile-bearing uncemented TAR has received FDA premarket conditional approval for use: the Scandinavian Total Ankle Replacement system (S.T.A.R. System, Small Bone Innovations, Inc, Morrisville, PA, USA/Stryker Orthopedics, Mahwah, NJ, USA).

The Agility Total Ankle Replacement System was the only US FDA–cleared ankle replacement readily available in the United States until 2007 (http://fda.gov/cdrh/panel/summary/ortho-04207.html; Accessed July 18, 2015). As a result, the Agility Total Ankle Replacement System was the most widely implanted ankle replacement in the United States for over a decade. It is well established that the Agility Total Ankle Replacement System was unforgiving as a primary prosthesis. A review of publications specific to the complication rate associated with primary implantation of the Agility Total Ankle Replacement System during the surgeon learning curve period reveals an incidence of complications of 60.8% (141/232).[4,7,14,15] The authors were able to further categorically divide these complications based on both the classification system proposed by Glazebrook and colleagues[16] and the simplified system proposed by Gadd and colleagues.[17] Under the classification system of Glazebrook and colleagues,[16] 14.2% of the complications were considered high grade, 29.1% were medium grade, and 50.3% were low grade. Under the classification system of Gadd and colleagues,[17] 43.3% were considered high grade, whereas 50.3% were low grade. According to each classification system, 6.4% of complications were unclassified, and these consisted of nerve and tendon injuries.

Although highly dependent on the specific TAR prosthesis system used, debate remains as to whether patients with failed primary TAR are best served with revision

TAR[18–27] or tibiotalocalcaneal (TTC) arthrodesis[28–30] most commonly using bulk intercalary allograft, although trabecular metal spacers are available for use outside the United States.[31] Although not definitive, a systematic review of the incidence of revision, defined as component replacement, ankle or TTC arthrodesis, or below-knee amputation (BKA)[32] after primary implantation of the uncemented Agility Total Ankle Replacement System was determined to be 10.2% (240 revisions/2353 primary implants) at a weighted mean follow-up of only 24.1 months.[15,33] Specifically, 78.6% of the revisions consisted of implant component replacement followed by arthrodesis (18.7% of revisions) and BKA (4.7% of revisions). Since the introduction of other TAR systems into the US market, the Agility Total Ankle Replacement System has fallen into disuse. The Agility LP Total Ankle Replacement System does not appear to have gained any traction since only one study involving clinical data exists. This lone unpublished US National Institutes of Health 2-year outcome study completed in 2012 involved 50 noncemented Agility LP Total Ankle Systems and revealed complications similar to the older Agility Total Ankle Replacement designs (Available at: http://www.clinicaltrials.gov/ct2/show/results/NCT01366872?term= ankle+replacement%27&rank=9&sect=X430125; Accessed July 18, 2015). The bulk of the volume of primary Agility Total Ankle Replacement Systems were implanted in the United States between 1998 and 2007 and the Agility LP Total Ankle Replacement System between 2007 and 2010. Therefore, it is reasonable to assume that surgeons unfamiliar with primary implantation of the Agility and Agility LP Total Ankle Replacement Systems will encounter patients with failure of these prostheses that would benefit from revision. To the authors' knowledge, there are no published data on the incidence of complications during revision of the Agility or Agility LP Total Ankle Replacement Systems during the surgeon learning curve period. Therefore, the authors sought to determine the incidence of complications in the intraoperative and early postoperative period during the senior author's learning curve period with revision of the Agility and Agility LP Total Ankle Replacement Systems.

MATERIALS AND METHODS

An observational case series was performed involving a retrospective review of prospectively collected data of the first 32 consecutive revision procedures performed by the senior author for the management of failed primary Agility and Agility LP Total Ankle Replacement Systems at the authors' facility between October 2010 and August 2014. The senior author is the director of the TAR surveillance program and inherited a practice that involved 192 primary implantations of the Agility and Agility LP Total Ankle Replacement Systems, including 68 (35.4%) original, 70 (36.5%) posterior augmented, 38 (19.8%) LP, and 16 (8.3%) revision talar components. All but one of the primary replacements in the series were performed by a single surgeon at the authors' facility before retiring, and the lone remaining replacement was performed by a different surgeon at an outside health care center. It should be noted that none of the primary Agility and Agility LP Total Ankle Replacement Systems had polymethylmethacrylate (PMMA) cement fixation, despite this being included in the surgeon technique guides.[34,35]

Each patient demonstrated varied severity of pathologic condition or persistent pain indicative of implant failure, but all were deemed to be at significant risk for impending catastrophic consequences if they elected not to undergo TAR revision. At the time of preoperative evaluation, based on comparison of serial weight-bearing radiographs over time, 18 of the 32 (56.3%) patients demonstrated progressive aseptic osteolysis of 5 mm or greater of the tibia predominantly about the medial malleolus or syndesmosis, fibula about the vertical lateral tibial component side wall, or talus predominantly within the neck region adjacent to the half pin used during external fixation application. Six of these were considered massive osteolysis of 15 mm or greater and involving cortical breach of the adjacent bone; 8 patients exhibited 5° or greater of progressive varus or valgus component malalignment; 3 patients were found to have clinically significant lateral ankle instability uncontrolled by prescription brace therapy; 2 patients had confirmed deep periprosthetic infection; 2 patients had obvious syndesmosis nonunion; and 1 patient presented with multiple periprosthetic midfoot fractures following a traumatic injury.[35] At the time of revision, 29 (90.6%) patients had documented talar component loosening with 8 (27.6%) of these patients also exhibiting loosening of the tibial component. Twenty-three patients (71.9%) underwent component revision of the ultrahigh-molecular-weight polyethylene (UHMWPE) insert and talar component to either a Revision or an LP design using the Agility or Agility LP Total Ankle Replacement Systems. Eight (25%) patients with massive osteolysis or severe 15° varus deformity or greater underwent explantation of the Agility Total Ankle Replacement System and conversion to the INBONE II Total Ankle Replacement System. One (3.2%) patient underwent explantation of the Agility Total Ankle Replacement System and conversion to the Salto Talaris XT Revision Ankle Prosthesis. **Table 1** highlights the details specific to each of these revision TAR procedures.

The authors use a standardized approach to the management of each revision TAR, allowing for deviation and augmentation to this approach on an individual basis as clinically required. In brief, they use a standard anterior ankle incision along the previous surgical incision, with careful soft tissue dissection to the level of the ankle joint capsule or scar, taking care to protect the anterior neurovascular bundle and maintain appropriate tissue planes for layered closure. Retraction is minimized to only what is necessary to aid in preservation of the tenuous anterior soft tissues.[41] Following entry into the ankle joint space and evacuation of the UHMWPE wear debris that is sent for histopathology, the periosteal tissues are elevated directly off the bone overlying the tibial component and then the talar component. Soft tissue exposure is limited to only what is needed to visualize the metallic components along with the medial and lateral gutters. Once soft tissue dissection is completed, the UHMWPE insert is removed by prying it free from the undersurface of the tibial tray. The talar component is freed from ectopic bone growth and then gently pried free of the underlying bone with care taken not to fracture the talus during manipulation. Although limited osseous ongrowth to the talar component was appreciated in each revision surgery regardless of talar component design, a consistent region where bonding did predictably occur was along the medial side of the keel. Accordingly, the authors recommend that great care be taken to liberate this region of the talar component from the talar bone followed by careful manipulation of the talar component during extirpation.

In the case of talar component exchange with retention of the tibial component, the remaining talar bone surface is prepared for implantation of the new talar component with care taken to correct any pre-existing osseous malalignment and to select the UHMWPE insert that will most appropriately tension the ankle joint ligamentous structures, which frequently involved redoing the talar keel after correcting the rotation and anterior-posterior alignment of the talar component for optimum function. The options for revision of the talar component depend on whether the failed system was an Agility or Agility LP Total Ankle Replacement System. The revision talar component adds between 1.5 mm and 2.8 mm of height (**Table 2**). In addition, several UHMWPE insert options exist depending on the specific version of the Agility or Agility LP Total Ankle

Table 1
Series patient population data (n = 32 ankles in 32 patients)

Case No.	DOS Index	Index TAR Specifics (Tibia/Talar Component; UHMWPE Insert)	DOS Revision	Revision TAR Specifics (Tibia/Talar Component; UHMWPE Insert)	Additional Procedures[36–40]	Age at Index TAR (y)	Age at Revision TAR (y)	Laterality (L/R)	Gender (M/F)	Complications
1	11/18/2008	3/3 LP; 0 mm	10/13/2010	No UHMWPE	—	78	81	L	M	—
2	2/22/2007	4/4 LP; 0 mm	5/20/2011	Custom stemmed 4 LP talar (+6 mm); 0 mm	—	72	77	R	M	—
3	9/25/2003	3/3 Revision; +2 mm	6/20/2011	Custom stemmed 3 LP talar (+8/+10 mm); +2 mm	—	36	44	R	F	—
4	3/31/1998	3/3 Original; 0 mm	10/7/2011	Custom stemmed 5 LP talar (+2 mm); custom stemmed 5 augmented tibial (+13.3 mm); +1 mm	Evans PB lateral ankle stabilization[36]	57	70	R	M	—
5	4/16/2009	2/2 LP; 0 mm	10/7/2011	Custom stemmed 2 LP talar (+3 mm); +2 mm	Evans PB lateral ankle stabilization[36]	53	55	L	F	—
6	12/19/1995	2/2 Original; 0 mm	3/23/2012	Conversion to INBONE II: 5 (18 mm base, 18 mm midstem, 16 mm midstem, 16 mm stem top)/ 4 talar dome, no stem; 10-mm size 4+	Intraoperative ORIF medial malleolus, fibula, and talus Fx	61	78	R	F	Intraoperative Fx; nonhealing incision with 2°BKA

(continued on next page)

Table 1
(continued)

Case No.	DOS Index	Index TAR Specifics (Tibia/Talar Component; UHMWPE Insert)	DOS Revision	Revision TAR Specifics (Tibia/Talar Component; UHMWPE Insert)	Additional Procedures[36–40]	Age at Index TAR (y)	Age at Revision TAR (y)	Laterality (L/R)	Gender (M/F)	Complications
7	8/9/2005	4/4 Original; +2 mm	5/4/2012	Conversion to INBONE II: 5 (18-mm base, 18-mm midstem, 16-mm midstem, 14-mm midstem, 14-mm stem top)/4 talar dome, 10-mm stem; 10-mm size 4+	Metal-reinforced PMMA augmentation tibia[37] and talus[38]	45	52	L	M	—
8	12/31/2003	5/5 Posterior augmented; 0 mm	6/15/2012	Conversion to INBONE II: 4 long (18-mm base, 18-mm midstem, 18-mm midstem, 16-mm midstem, 16-mm midstem, 14-mm stem top)/3 talar dome, 10-mm stem; 10-mm size 3+	Intraoperative ORIF medial malleolus and fibula Fx	59	68	R	M	Intraoperative Fx; dorsal foot neuritis
9	3/25/2004	3/3 Posterior augmented; 0 mm	7/27/2012	3 Revision; ½ column 0 mm	ORIF traumatic navicular Fx, cuneiform Fx, and cuboid Fx	60	68	L	F	—

#	Date		Date							
10	1/17/2006	2/2 Revision; 0 mm	8/3/2012	Conversion to INBONE II: 5 long (18-mm base, 16-mm midstem, 14-mm midstem, 14-mm midstem, 14-mm midstem, 12-mm stem top)/5 talar dome, 14-mm stem; 13-mm size 5	Metal-reinforced PMMA[37,38]; superficial peroneal neurectomy with muscle implantation	43	49	L	M	—
11	8/20/2002	4/4 Posterior augmented; 0 mm	9/7/2012	4 Revision; +2 mm	Metal-reinforced PMMA tibia[37]; PMMA cement talus	70	80	L	M	—
12	3/26/2009	4/4 LP; 0 mm	10/26/2012	4 Revision; 0 mm	Metal-reinforced PMMA[37,38] syndesmosis; PB to PL transfer	66	69	L	M	—
13	2/4/2003	4/4 Posterior augmented; 0 mm	10/26/2012	4 Revision; $\frac{1}{2}$ column 0 mm	Metal-reinforced PMMA tibia[37] and talus[38]; PT recession[39], deltoid release	66	75	R	M	—
14	4/25/2006	4/4 Posterior augmented; 0 mm	11/23/2012	Conversion to INBONE II: 4 (18-mm base, 18-mm midstem, 16-mm midstem, 16-mm midstem, 14-mm midstem, 14 stem top)/3 talar dome, no stem; 10-mm size 3+	Metal-reinforced PMMA tibia[37] and talus[38]; intraoperative ORIF medial malleolus Fx	47	55	L	M	Intraoperative Fx

(continued on next page)

Table 1
(continued)

Case No.	DOS Index	Index TAR Specifics (Tibia/Talar Component; UHMWPE Insert)	DOS Revision	Revision TAR Specifics (Tibia/Talar Component; UHMWPE Insert)	Additional Procedures[36-40]	Age at Index TAR (y)	Age at Revision TAR (y)	Laterality (L/R)	Gender (M/F)	Complications
15	2/8/2007	3/3 LP; 0 mm	1/11/2013	4 Revision; mismatch 3/4	Metal-reinforced PMMA tibia[37]; Evans PB lateral ankle stabilization[36], PT recession[39]	67	73	R	M	Delayed incision healing
16	9/23/2009	6/6 LP; 0 mm	1/18/2013	6 Revision; +1 mm	Metal-reinforced PMMA tibia[37] and syndesmosis; PB to PL transfer	61	64	L	M	—
17	9/14/2004	4/4 Posterior augmented; 0 mm	1/25/2013	4 LP; +2 mm	Metal-reinforced PMMA tibia[37] and syndesmosis; Evans PB lateral ankle stabilization[36]	58	67	R	M	—
18	7/1/2003	5/5 Revision; 0 mm	3/8/2013	5 LP; +2 mm	Metal-reinforced PMMA tibia[37]	66	76	R	M	—
19	10/21/1999	4/4 Original; 0 mm	3/22/2013	4 LP; +2 mm	—	32	46	L	F	—
20	6/20/2011	3 LP custom stemmed posterior augmented talar (+8/+10 mm); +2 mm	3/22/2013	Conversion to INBONE II: 4 (18-mm base, 14-mm stem top)/ 4 talar dome, 14-mm stem; 15-mm size 4	Reverse Evans PB deltoid reconstruction[40]	36	46	L	F	—

21	11/7/2002	5/5 Posterior augmented; 0 mm	4/19/2013	5 Revision; +2 mm	Metal-reinforced PMMA talus[38]	63	74	L	M	—
22	8/3/2006	5/5 Posterior augmented; 0 mm	5/31/2013	5 LP; +2 mm	Metal-reinforced PMMA fibula and talus[38]; Evans PB lateral ankle stabilization[36], PL to PB tendon transfer; PTT recession[39], deltoid release	56	63	L	M	—
23	4/25/2008	4/4 LP; 0 mm	5/31/2013	5 LP; mismatch 4/5	Metal-reinforced PMMA talus[38]	68	73	L	M	—
24	3/18/2003	3/3 Posterior augmented; 0 mm	6/7/2013	3 LP; +2 mm	Metal-reinforced PMMA talus[38]	62	72	R	F	—
25	2/6/2009	3 tibia LP; 4 LP talus; mismatch 3/4	8/9/2013	3 Revision; 0 mm	—	62	66	R	F	Delayed incision healing
26	7/8/2004	3/3 LP; 0 mm	8/23/2013	3 LP; +2 mm	Evans PB lateral ankle stabilization[36]	39	48	L	F	—
27	2/1/2007	4/4 LP; 0 mm	8/30/2013	4 LP; +1 mm	Metal-reinforced PMMA tibia[37]	42	48	R	F	—
28	3/27/2008	4/4 LP; 0 mm	11/20/2013	4 LP; 0 mm	Metal-reinforced PMMA tibia[37]	51	56	L	M	—

(continued on next page)

Table 1
(continued)

Case No.	DOS Index	Index TAR Specifics (Tibia/Talar Component; UHMWPE Insert)	DOS Revision	Revision TAR Specifics (Tibia/Talar Component; UHMWPE Insert)	Additional Procedures[36–40]	Age at Index TAR (y)	Age at Revision TAR (y)	Laterality (L/R)	Gender (M/F)	Complications
29	10/7/2008	4/4 LP; 0 mm	11/29/2013	Conversion to INBONE II: 4 long (18-mm base, 16-mm midstem, 16-mm stem top)/3 talar dome, 10-mm stem; 10-mm size 3+	PTT recession[39]; deltoid release; tarsal tunnel release; PB Evans lateral ankle stabilization[36]. TAL	56	61	L	M	—
30	12/11/2008	4/4 LP; 0 mm	12/6/2013	Conversion to INBONE II: 5 (18-mm base, 16-mm midstem, 14-mm midstem, 12-mm midstem, 12-mm stem top)/5 talar dome, 10-mm stem; 15-mm size 5	Intraoperative ORIF medial malleolus Fx	52	57	L	M	Intraoperative Fx
31	8/14/2008	5/5 LP; 0 mm	1/31/2014	6 LP; mismatch 5/6	Metal-reinforced PMMA syndesmosis; reverse Evans PB deltoid reconstruction[40], 1st MTPJ arthrodesis	73	79	L	M	—
32	11/8/2005	3/3 Posterior augmented; 0 mm	8/8/2014	Conversion to 2/2 Salto Talaris XT; 5 mm (Th 9)	Metal-reinforced PMMA tibia[37]/fibula; deltoid release; TAL	69	78	L	F	—

Agility Total Ankle Replacement (DePuy Synthes Joint Reconstruction); INBONE II Total Ankle Replacement (Wright Medical Technology, Inc); Salto Talaris XT Revision Ankle Prosthesis (Tornier).

Abbreviations: DOS, date of surgery; F, female; Fx, fracture; L, left; LP, low profile; M, male; MTPJ, metatarsophalangeal joint; NCJ, naviculocuneiform joint; ORIF, open reduction internal fixation; PB, peroneus brevis; PL, peroneus longus; PMMA, polymethylmethacrylate cement; PTT, posterior tibialis tendon; R, right; TA, tibialis anterior; TAL, percutaneous tendo-Achilles lengthening.

Table 2
Specific height dimensions for the Agility Revision and LP Total Ankle Replacement System talar components

Size	UHMWPE Insert				
	0 mm	+1 mm	Mismatch (mm)	LP Talar (mm)	Revision Talar (mm)
1	3.7	4.7	3.7	11.8	13.3
2	3.7	4.7	3.7	12.3	14.1
3	3.9	4.9	3.9	12.8	14.9
4	3.9	4.9	3.9	13.1	15.7
5	3.9	4.9	3.9	14.1	16.9
6	4.6	5.7	3.9	15.6	17.8

Note. The original Agility Total Ankle Replacement system original talar component and posterior augmented have the same height specifics as the Agility LP talar component.

Replacement System undergoing revision as follows. If the failed system is an Agility Total Ankle Replacement System, then the revision options include (1) same size revision talar component with bottom-loaded full or one-half column 0-mm UHMWPE insert; (2) same size revision talar component with bottom-loaded full column + 2-mm UHMWPE insert; or (3) same size LP talar component with bottom-loaded full column + 2-mm UHMWPE insert. If the failed system is an Agility LP Total Ankle Replacement System, then the revision options include (1) same size revision talar component with front-loaded 0-mm UHMWPE insert; (2) same size revision talar component with front-loaded + 1-mm UHMWPE insert; (3) same size LP talar component with front-loaded 0-mm UHMWPE insert (note that this is only possible if the talar component subsidence is corrected back to its original state with the use of PMMA cement augmentation; otherwise, an unstable joint will result); (4) same size LP talar component with front-loaded + 1-mm UHMWPE insert; (5) one size larger revision talar component with front-loaded mismatch UHMWPE insert (ie, retained size 4 LP tibial tray with size 5 revision talar component and size 5/4 mismatch UHMWPE insert); and (6) one size larger LP talar component with front-loaded mismatch UHMWPE insert. It should be noted that the mismatch UHMWPE insert does not independently add any additional height.[34,38] When varus deformities persisted after osseous preparation of the talus to correct the malalignment, a posterior tibial tendon recession was performed at the musculotendinous junction[39]; furthermore, a deep deltoid release off the talus was carried out if additional correction was required.

Regardless of the components implanted, liberal use of intraoperative C-arm image intensification is used to confirm adequate osseous preparation and metallic component position. If the varus ankle was coupled with lateral ankle instability, this was corrected with an extra-anatomic autogenous peroneus brevis tendon transfer to the distal-lateral tibia to achieve lateral ligament reconstruction.[36] Similarly, when valgus deformities were encountered, osseous preparation of the talus to correct any malalignment was performed. If the valgus ankle was coupled with medial ankle instability, this was corrected with an extra-anatomic autogenous peroneus brevis tendon through the talar neck and secured to the distal medial tibia for deltoid reconstruction.[40] Beyond these mentioned, the authors did not encounter the need to perform other osseous osteotomy, arthrodesis, or tendon balancing procedures to achieve a balanced ankle.

In the event of explantation and conversion to a different TAR system, the appropriate technique per the specific TAR system is followed.[22,26,27,42] For each revision, the authors chose to use a thin layer of antibiotic-impregnated PMMA cement (Simplex P with Tobramycin; Stryker Orthopedics) about the perimeter of the replaced metallic components when good osseous apposition was possible. In situations involving advanced aseptic osteolysis and resultant contained osseous defects from cyst formation, they used metal-reinforced antibiotic-impregnated PMMA cement to backfill the osseous defect and secondarily provide some early stability to the metallic components.[38,39,43]

It should be noted that in order to reduce the potential for deep periprosthetic infection, traffic about and number of people in the operating room are kept to an absolute minimum. For the week immediately preceding the surgery, patients perform a daily 5-minute scrub of their surgical limb with chlorhexidine gluconate (4%) solution (Hibiclens; Regent Medical Americas, Norcross, GA, USA). In addition, the authors perform a validated surgical preparation involving the foot, ankle, and lower leg using a 3-minute scrub with foam sponges impregnated with chlorhexidine gluconate (4%) solution followed by painting with ethyl alcohol and iodine (1%) topical solution (1 g iodine/100 mL ethyl alcohol) (Spectrum Chemical Manufacturing Corporation, Gardena, CA; USA).[44] Furthermore, the toes are covered with an impermeable incise barrier; the exposed skin is intermittently repainted with Betadine Solution (10% povidone iodine solution; Purdue Products, LP, Stamford, CT, USA), and the surgical site is serially irrigated with a pulsed lavage system impregnated with 50,000 IU Bacitracin solution (Pfizer, Inc, New York, NY, USA) per 3-L bag. The operating rooms are all laminar flow systems without ultraviolet lights. Each member of the surgical team wears double surgical masks or a surgical hood/space suit based on personal preference.

If deep periprosthetic infection was present at the time of revision, in addition to the above, the authors performed extensive debridement of the entire intra-articular soft tissues and bone with a hydrosurgery device (Versajet II; Smith & Nephew Advanced Wound Management, Hull, UK) until only healthy bleeding tissues remained. The authors used Gentamycin solution (320 mg) and Tobramycin powder (2.4 g) antibiotic-loaded PMMA cement beads and negative pressure wound therapy (V.A.C. Therapy; Kinetic Concepts, Inc, San Antonio, TX, USA) to reduce edema and function as a mechanical leech. Serial operative sessions including high-volume irrigation, debridement, and antibiotic-loaded PMMA cement bead exchange were performed every 48 hours until no further clinical or microbiological evidence of persistent infection was evident. Revision TAR was then performed using the principles above. Parenteral culture-specific antibiotics managed by an infectious disease specialist were undertaken for 6 weeks along with an extended course of oral antibiotic therapy for an additional 3 months.

Meticulous, layered closure is essential. Every patient receives a surgical drain and an anterior windowed folded Webril Undercast Padding (Kendall-Coviden, Mansfield, MA, USA) cut out to the anterior incision line (**Fig. 1**) with additional Sir Robert Jones compression dressing and posterior molded plaster splint. The authors have found that the anterior windowed folded Webril Undercast Padding limits contact pressure on the tenuous anterior incision and the Sir Robert Jones dressing affords edema reduction during the postoperative period.[45] All patients follow the standard postoperative protocol for TAR as previously described.[46,47] In brief, this protocol includes hospital admission, 48 hours of intravenous antibiotic therapy with a first-generation cephalosporin, strict bed rest protocol with lower extremities elevated above heart level and heels offloaded using pillow cocoon, and a semi-Fowler bed-positioning protocol. Although anecdotal, supplemental oxygen via nasal cannula during the hospitalization is routinely used because it may reduce incision and ischemia-related wound-healing problems. The patients' activities with physical and occupational

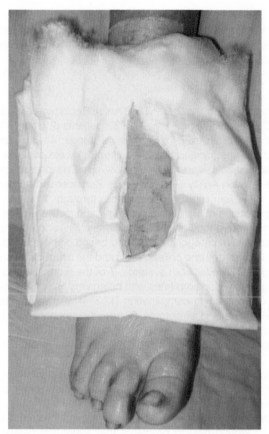

Fig. 1. Clinical photograph of the anterior aspect of the ankle following revision TAR demonstrating a nonstick dressing deep to a layered anterior windowed folded Webril Undercast Padding (Kendall-Coviden) cut out to the anterior incision line.

therapy are advanced while maintaining strict non-weight-bearing to the operative lower extremity and discharge to home versus a skilled nursing facility proceeds. Patients are maintained on a strict mechanical and pharmacologic thromboembolic prophylaxis protocol until a return to full weight-bearing and activity is realized. At the 8-week follow-up appointment, weight-bearing ankle radiographs are obtained and, if no complications are noted, patients are permitted to transition into full weight-bearing and back into a supportive shoe or lace-up high-topped boot. Weight-bearing ankle radiographs are obtained including stress sagittal plane dorsiflexion and plantarflexion as well as long leg axial[48] views 1 year from the revision TAR and every year thereafter during the annual surveillance program used by the senior author. Although controversial, dental antibiotic prophylaxis, use of a brace or lace-up high-topped boot with any exposure to uneven ground, and avoidance of ballistic activities are enforced lifelong.

The senior author uses the New Zealand Joint Registry Revision Ankle Joint data form (http://www.nzoa.org.nz/system/files/NJR%2014%20Year%20Report.pdf; page 135; Accessed July 18, 2015) to record all patient demographics and specifics associated with revision TAR. All complications associated with the TAR revision procedure were documented as they occurred. Following each revision TAR, the senior author performed an interim analysis of all revision TAR procedures performed to determine the cause of any complications encountered in order to limit a negative trend with subsequent patients.

RESULTS

A total of 32-revision Agility or Agility LP Total Ankle Replacement System procedures (20 left ankles, 12 right ankles) performed on 32 patients (21 men, 11 women) with a mean age at the time of revision of 64.6 years (range: 44–81 years) and a mean follow-up of 25.6 months (range: 12.2–50.4 months) were evaluated for this study (see **Table 1**). No patients were lost to follow-up. One patient died of unrelated reasons than the revision Agility LP Total Ankle Replacement surgery at 30 months postoperatively; however, regular surveillance through 2 years postoperatively revealed no complications of the revision surgery, and thus, the patient was included in the review. There were a total of 8 complications (25%) encountered (see **Table 1**). These complications were categorically divided based on both the classification system proposed by Glazebrook and colleagues[16] and the simplified system proposed by Gadd and colleagues.[17] Under both systems, 7 of the 8 complications (87.5%) were classified as low grade, which correlates with being very unlikely to cause subsequent TAR failure.[16,17] The remaining complication (12.5%) was unclassified and involved unresolved dorsal foot neuritic symptoms. Of note, no complications were considered high grade or medium grade, which would correlate with a likelihood of leading to failure of the implant 50% of the time or more or less than 50% of the time, respectively.[16,17]

The authors also compared the results of the first 16 patients with the next 16, during the senior author's learning curve period for revision Agility or Agility LP Total Ankle Replacement (**Table 3**). Six of the 8 complications (75%) occurred in the early group, whereas only 2 complications (25%) occurred in the late group, both of which consisted of minor wound-healing problems that eventually healed conservatively. The overall incidence of complications occurring in the early group was 37.5% (6/16), which decreased by two-thirds in the late group, to 12.5% (2/16) (see **Table 3**).

DISCUSSION

The purpose of this study was to determine the incidence of complications in the intraoperative and early postoperative period during the senior author's learning curve period with revision Agility or Agility LP Total Ankle Replacement as well as to compare these results with those identified for primary Agility or Agility LP Total Ankle Replacement during the surgeon learning period. This case series involved the first 32 consecutive revision Agility or Agility LP Total Ankle Replacements performed by the senior author and yielded an overall incidence of complications of 25%, with most complications occurring in the early group of patients. The incidence of low-grade complications according to the classification systems of Glazebrook and colleagues[16] and of Gadd and colleagues[17] was 21.9%, and the incidence of unclassified complications (ie, nerve damage) was 3.1%. There were no high- or medium-grade complications in this series. Once again, according to data compiled by the authors, the incidence of complications associated with primary implantation of the Agility Total Ankle Replacement System during the surgeon learning curve was 60.8% (141/232).[4,7,14,15] Under the classification system of Glazebrook and colleagues,[16] 14.2% of these complications were considered high grade, 29.1% were medium grade, and 50.3% were low grade. Under the classification system of Gadd and colleagues,[17]

Table 3
Comparison of complications in early versus late group

Patient Group (Early/Late)	Case No.	Revision TAR Procedure	No. of Complications	Complication Details	Glazebrook[16]/ Gadd[17] Classification
Early	6	Conversion to INBONE II	2	Intraoperative Fx; nonhealing incision with 2°BKA	Low; low
	8	Conversion to INBONE II	2	Intraoperative Fx; persistent dorsal foot neuritic symptoms	Low; unclassified
	14	Conversion to INBONE II	1	Intraoperative Fx	Low
	15	Agility to agility Revision Talar Component; mismatch 3/4 UHMWPE	1	Delayed incision healing	Low
Late	25	Agility to Agility Revision Talar Component; 0-mm UHMWPE	1	Delayed incision healing	Low
	30	Conversion to INBONE II	1	Intraoperative Fx	Low

Agility and Agility LP Total Ankle Replacement (DePuy Synthes Joint Reconstruction); INBONE II Total Ankle Replacement (Wright Medical Technology, Inc).
Abbreviation: Fx, fracture.

43.3% were considered high grade, whereas 50.3% were low grade. According to each classification system, 6.4% of complications were unclassified. Comparison of the revision Agility or Agility LP Total Ankle Replacement results from the authors' series to the primary Agility Total Ankle Replacement suggests that revision of these specific TAR systems during the surgeon learning period can be accomplished safely when performed meticulously by a qualified foot and ankle surgeon.

In addition to assessing the incidence of complications, the authors compared their data to the New Zealand Joint Registry Data, which was possible given that they document all patient data according to the New Zealand Joint Registry Revision Ankle Joint data form (http://www.nzoa.org.nz/system/files/NJR%2014%20Year%20Report.pdf; pages 108 and 109; Accessed July 18, 2015). For the 13-year period included in the 2013 New Zealand Joint Registry Data (January 2000 to December 2012),[49] there were 101 revision TAR procedures registered, of which 16 involved the Agility Total Ankle Replacement System. Unfortunately, the specific information associated with these revisions is not available (**Table 4**).

Another comparison the authors investigated within their series was between the 4 different categories of revision TAR procedures performed (**Table 5**). Specifically, of the 32 Agility and Agility LP Total Ankle Replacement Systems revisions, 19 (59.4%) were treated with Revision or LP talar component and UHMWPE revision; 8 (25%) with explantation and conversion to the INBONE II Total Ankle Replacement System; 3 (9.4%) with custom-designed stemmed Agility LP talar components with concomitant subtalar joint arthrodesis and UHMWPE revision; 1 (3.1%) with explantation and custom-designed stemmed Agility LP tibia and talar components with concomitant subtalar joint arthrodesis and UHMWPE revision; and 1 (3.1%) with explantation and conversion to the Salto Talaris XT Revision Ankle Prosthesis. Although only 2 (8.7%) complications occurred in the larger group undergoing Agility and Agility LP

Table 4
Data comparison of current series to the New Zealand Joint Registry

	New Zealand Joint Registry (2014)	Current Series
Period of Data Collection		
Months	168	46
Range	01/2000–12/2013	10/2010–08/2014
No. of Revisions		
Overall Number of TAR Revisions	101	32
Agility or Agility LP TAR requiring Revision	16	32
Age (y)		
Mean	64.8	64.6
Range	40.2–83.1	44–81
Gender (No.)		
Female	37	11
Male	64	21
Time to Revision (mo)		
Mean	43.5	78.7
Min	0.7	9.4
Max	156.1	195.1
SD	33.3	45.4
Reason for Revision		
Pain	37	16
Loosening Talar Component	22	29
Loosening Tibial Component	16	8
Deep infection	5	2

Agility and Agility LP Total Ankle Replacement Systems (DePuy Synthes Joint Reconstruction, Warsaw, IN).

Abbreviations: No., number; SD, standard deviation; TAR, total ankle replacement.

and custom-designed stemmed Total Ankle Replacement revision, 6 (75%) complications occurred in the explantation and conversion to INBONE II Total Ankle Replacement System group. This finding is significant because some authors have questioned the efficacy of revision TAR using the Agility Total Ankle Replacement Systems[50]; however, the authors' data suggest this is the much safer option when possible, as compared with total explantation and conversion to the INBONE II Total Ankle Replacement System. This concept of talar component and UHMWPE revision for failed primary Agility Total Ankle Replacement System implantation is an established, albeit somewhat historical approach to this vexing problem. As stated previously, a systematic review of the incidence of revision for failed primary uncemented Agility Total Ankle Replacement System prostheses was determined to be 10.2% (240 revisions/2353 primary implants) at a weighted mean follow-up of only 24.1 months.[15,33] Specifically, 78.6% (189/240) of the revisions performed consisted of implant component replacement. Regardless, the concept of talar component and UHMWPE revision approach has been extensively advocated in the literature,[15,18,20–22,34,39,42,43,51–56] but unfortunately, the only available published data involve 27 talar or tibial implant component replacements, of which 20 (74%) were considered to have had good or excellent outcomes at 24 months postoperatively.[18] In addition, at present, limited

Table 5
Comparison of Revision Agility and Agility LP Total Ankle Replacement options

	Patients at Revision (N)	Mean Age (y) (Range)	Gender	Laterality	Total Complications (N)	Incidence of Complications (%)	Early Complications (N)	Late Complications (N)	Mean Overall Operating Time (h:min)	Early Mean Operating Time (h:min)	Late Mean Operating Time (h:min)
Agility to Agility	19	67.3 (46–81)	13 M; 6 F	7 R; 12 L	2	8.7	1	1	3:27	3:49	3:08
Agility to Agility Custom-designed stemmed	4	61.5 (44–77)	2 M; 2 F	3 R; 1 L	0	0	0	0	4:51	4:51	—
Agility to INBONE II	8	58.3 (46–78)	6 M; 2 F	2 R; 6 L	6	75	3	2	6:14	6:27	6:02
Agility to Salto Talaris XT	1	78	1 F	1 L	0	0	0	0	3:49	—	—

Agility and Agility LP Total Ankle Replacement (DePuy Synthes Joint Reconstruction); INBONE II Total Ankle Replacement (Wright Medical Technology, Inc); Salto Talaris XT Revision Ankle Prosthesis (Tornier).

Abbreviations: F, female; L, left; M, male; R, right.

component availability for revision of the Agility or Agility LP Total Ankle Replacement is a very real problem. The Agility Total Ankle Replacement Original and Posterior Augmented talar components as well as the Agility LP Total Ankle Replacement Tibial Tray are no longer being manufactured. Furthermore, the Agility Total Ankle Replacement Revision and LP talar components along with UHMWPE inserts are in limited supply, essentially functioning as legacy products. These facts foretell the end of the Agility and Agility LP Total Ankle Replacement Systems for primary TAR and thus complicate revision options. Taken as a whole, the concept of talar component and UHMWPE revision for the management of the failed primary Agility and Agility LP Total Ankle Replacement Systems may have limited applicability in the future. Instead, alternative component revision strategies consisting of custom-designed stemmed tibial or talar components[42,54,57–59] or explantation and conversion to an alternative TAR system, specifically the INBONE II Total Ankle Replacement System[26,27,34] and Salto Talaris Total Ankle Prosthesis[21,22] or Salto Talaris XT Revision Ankle Prosthesis (Tornier, Inc), will be needed.

Of an original pool of 53 patients with failed primary Agility Total Ankle Replacement System, Ellington and colleagues[42] were able to evaluate 41 patients following revision at a mean follow-up of 49.1 months (range: 25.9–77.8 months). Revision consisted of talar component replacement only in 36.6% (15/41) and both tibial and talar component replacement in 63.4% (26/41). Of the entire cohort, 4.9% (2/41) underwent custom-designed stemmed tibial component replacement and 41.5% (19/41) underwent custom-designed stemmed talar component replacement with concomitant subtalar joint arthrodesis. The authors provided a grading system from 1 to 3 to define the severity of talar component subsidence and predict outcome following revision. In grade 1, there is minimal subsidence of the talar component. In grade 2, the talar component has subsided into the talar body but has not violated the subtalar joint. Grade 3 is where the talar component has migrated onto or through the subtalar joint. Using a multivariable linear regression analysis, preoperative talar subsidence was a significant predictor of a good outcome following revision. Based on these results, McCollum and Myerson[22] concluded that the revision options for grade 1 and early grade 2 talar component subsidence involving the Agility Total Ankle Replacement System are to use the Revision or LP talar components. For severe subsidence associated with late grade 2 and grade 3 or with anticipated inability of the talus to support a Revision or LP talar component, the use of a custom-designed stemmed talar component is recommended.[22,42] The authors had 4 patients who underwent conversion to custom-designed stemmed LP talar components and concomitant subtalar joint arthrodesis with one of these, including a custom-designed stemmed tibial component. Three of the 4 have done well clinically, and none of these had complications intraoperatively or postoperatively. One of the custom-designed stemmed talar components underwent progressive component migration and subsequently required explantation and conversion to an INBONE II Total Ankle Replacement System. Unfortunately, as of December 8, 2011, any Agility or Agility LP Total Ankle Replacement System custom-designed stemmed talar component is no longer available for clinical use due to US FDA regulation, and the availability of this in the future remains uncertain (http://www.fda.gov/ICECI/EnforcementActions/WarningLetters/2011/ucm287552.htm; Accessed July 18, 2015). It should be noted that the complexity of revision Agility Total Ankle Replacement is borne out by the fact that Ellington and colleagues,[42] who were experienced with primary implantation of the Agility and Agility LP Total Ankle Replacement Systems, required further revision in the form of TTC arthrodesis in 12.2% (5/41) for progressive component migration with subsidence and BKA in 4.9% (2/41) as a complication of deep periprosthetic infection. Myerson and colleagues[60] presented an incidence of deep periprosthetic infection following primary Agility and Agility LP Total Ankle Replacement Systems of 3.2% (14/433) compared with 0.7% (1/139) following primary Salto Talaris Total Ankle Prosthesis implantation. The authors did not encounter the development of a deep periprosthetic infection after revision TAR in their patient population to date. However, it seems that a major concern for both primary and revision Agility and Agility LP Total Ankle Replacement is deep periprosthetic infection, and efforts to minimize infection, such as the protocol used by the senior author, should be diligently followed. The mean clinical follow-up of patients was 25.6 months (range: 12.2–50.4 months), and during this period, they did not encounter a failure of the revision surgery performed. However, the authors' results cannot be directly compared with those of Ellington and colleagues [42] because the authos focused on the incidence of complications encountered with revision of failed primary Agility and Agility LP Total Ankle Replacement Systems and not clinical outcomes over time.

Explantation of the failed Agility and Agility LP Total Ankle Replacement Systems with conversion to the INBONE II Total Ankle Replacement System has been reported previously and is considered a limb-salvage procedure. DeVries et al[26] reported an overall incidence of complications of 64.3% (9/14) for the 13 conversions performed through an anterior incision and one through a posterior incision. The mean age at time of revision was 65.2 years (range: 45–79 years) for the 8 men and 6 women included. The Agility Total Ankle Replacement System had been in place a mean of 7.8 years (range: 3.5–23 years). Based on the presented details of each of the 9 complications, the authors were able to categorize them according to the classification systems of Glazebrook and colleagues[16] and of Gadd and colleagues.[17] According to Glazebrook and colleagues,[16] 2 of the 9 complications (22.2%) were high grade and both involved deep infection, 1 (11.1%) was medium grade consisting of malposition necessitating secondary alignment procedures, and 1 (11.1%) was low grade involving minor wounding. The remaining 5 complications (55.6%) were unclassified and involved the need for secondary neurolysis, minor asymptomatic subsidence, and "residual pain." According to Gadd and colleagues,[17] the same complications were categorized as 3 high grade (33.3%), 1 low grade (11.1%), and 5 unclassified (55.6%). The authors' results compare favorably with no incidence of high- or medium-grade complications as well as fewer unclassified complications. Meeker and colleagues[27] reported an overall incidence of complications of 27.7% (5/18) for the 18 conversions performed through an anterior incision. The original Agility Total Ankle Replacement System had been in place a mean of 12.8 years (range: 1.6–13.4 years). As with the previously discussed article, based on the presented details, the authors categorized each of the 5 complications reported by Meeker and colleagues[27] according to the classification systems of Glazebrook and colleagues[16] and of Gadd and colleagues.[17] According to Glazebrook and colleagues,[16] 1 of the 5 complications (20%) was considered medium grade and involved postoperative dislocation of the prosthesis, while 3 (60%) were low grade consisting of intraoperative fractures. According to Gadd and colleagues,[17] the postoperative prosthetic dislocation would be classified as high grade (20%), whereas the 3 intraoperative fractures would remain classified as low grade (60%). The remaining complication (20%) was unclassified per both systems and involved posterior tibial nerve compression that required neurolysis. The results are more comparable with those of Meeker and colleagues[27]; however, once again, the authors report no high-grade complications according to either the classification system of Glazebrook and colleagues[16] or the classification system of Gadd and colleagues.[17]

Another interesting comparison between the revision groups in the authors' series included the mean operating time (ie, skin incision to final closure) (see **Table 5**). The Agility and Agility LP Total Ankle Replacement Systems exchange group had a mean ± standard deviation operating time of 3 hours and 27 minutes ± 1 hour and 6 minutes. Meanwhile, the conversion to INBONE II Total Ankle Replacement System group had a mean ± standard deviation operating time of 6 hours and 14 minutes ± 52 minutes. This clinically significant difference in operating time, combined with the much more frequent incidence of complications, demonstrates the sheer complexity and incredible demands required of a foot and ankle surgeon performing revision for failed Agility and Agility LP Total Ankle Replacement Systems with explantation and conversion to the INBONE II Total Ankle Replacement System. Alternatively, although only performed once at the time of writing this article, the authors found that explantation of a failed Agility Total Ankle Replacement System and conversion to the Salto Talaris XT Revision Ankle Prosthesis was technically easier than conversion to the INBONE II Total Ankle Replacement System. This isolated case took 3 hours and 49 minutes to complete and was devoid of complications. The Salto Talaris XT Revision Ankle Prosthesis consists of size 1, 2, and 3 talar components containing a flat cut and longer peg and 9-, 11-, 13-mm-thick revision UHMWPE inserts with additional 15- and 17-mm-thick inserts being projected for use by mid-2015 (Note that the mm-thicknesses described are the actual thicknesses not the Th listed by the manufacturer). The tibial components are the same as the size 1, 2, and 3 Salto Talaris Total Ankle Prosthesis, but a stemmed tibial component with a long central keel is projected to be available for use by mid-2015 and is currently available for use in the United States by surgeon prescription only on a compassionate use basis. The ability for the Salto Talaris XT Revision Ankle Prosthesis to revise failed Agility and Agility LP Total Ankle Replacement Systems is certainly intriguing but currently unproven.

Taking the published reports and the current data into account, although revision of failed primary Agility and Agility Total Ankle Replacement Systems with talar component and UHMWPE insert revision is not the universal option, when appropriate, it is certainly a viable option given the greater safety as compared with explantation and conversion to the INBONE II Total Ankle Replacement System. Clearly, a real need exists for outcome studies to evaluate patients undergoing explantation and conversion revision TAR for the current prosthesis systems available in the United States, and future efforts should be directed in this area.

The outcomes of revised primary Agility and Agility LP Total Ankle Replacement Systems regardless of approach deserves additional investigation because the potential does exist that, rather than implant component replacement, it would be more prudent to perform arthrodesis for failure of these particular TAR systems. However, at present, this remains a matter for conjecture, because the data available demonstrate that revision surgery consists predominantly of implant component revision and not arthrodesis for the Agility and Agility LP Total Ankle Replacement Systems. The authors contend that, when possible, talar component and UHMWPE insert revision with the addition of reinforcement of contained osseous defects using antibiotic-impregnated PMMA cement with or without metal augmentation[34,39,40,43] is the procedure selection of choice. Explantation with conversion to the Salto Talaris XT Revision Ankle Prosthesis is a viable option when limited bone loss exists, but until thicker UHMPWE inserts and stemmed tibial components are readily available, it remains underpowered for universal use with revision of the failed Agility and Agility LP Total Ankle Replacement Systems. Explantation with conversion to the INBONE II Total Ankle Replacement as a "megaprosthesis" is warranted when other options are not feasible, and the osseous defect is massive such that even TTC with bulk intercalary allograft would be challenging. As the data and previously published reports support, the surgeon and patient should expect a high incidence of complications to occur with this approach. Before using the INBONE II Total Ankle Replacement, the preferred method of revision for situations with critical tibial or talar bone loss was custom-designed stemmed Agility LP tibial or talar components because restoration of tibial or talar height was unlimited and the long stems provided sound support as well as a large surface for osseous ongrowth. The authors maintain and the literature supports that, although not currently available for use in the United States, custom-designed stemmed TAR components represent viable options and should also be relevant in the future once the FDA loosens the current restrictions. Revision INBONE I Total Ankle Replacement with the talar component supported by metal-reinforced triangular rods and large-diameter screws affixed within a PMMA cement mantle,[61] permanent PMMA cement spacer,[60,62] TTC arthrodesis with bulk intercalary allograft,[28–30] or BKA[28] should be reserved for select non-reconstructable cases, uncontrollable deep periprosthetic infection, or situations wherein the patient does not desire or is medically unable to undergo revision surgery.

In addition to the comments above, several more weaknesses of this study were considered. First, the authors used 2 yet-to-be validated classifications systems designed to categorize complications associated with primary TAR during the surgeon learning curve period and assess the likelihood of implant failure as a means of classifying the complications associated with revision of failed primary Agility and Agility Total Ankle Replacement Systems. Although the classification system of Glazebrook and colleagues[16] involved a large portion of Agility Total Ankle Replacement Systems, the classification system of Gladd and colleagues[17] did not. In addition, neither classification system has been validated. Therefore, the prognostic value of these systems on predicting future failure of the revised Agility and Agility Total Ankle Replacement Systems remains unanswered. However, these are the currently available classification systems, and in general, very similar risks of complications exist in both primary and revision TAR regardless of the specific prosthetic components used. Furthermore, both classification systems yielded the same number and category of complications for the data. The authors' follow-up criteria were a bit lenient since we did not use, given the authors included a patient less than 1 month postoperatively from their revision, and they did not use any validated patient outcomes-related scoring scale to determine how successful the revision TAR procedures were from the patient perspective. However, the primary goal of this study was to assess complications in the intraoperative and early postoperative period, not patient satisfaction and function, although thus far, none of the included patients exhibit signs of impending complication. Finally, the effect of the senior author's protocol on the incidence of complications encountered during the intraoperative and perioperative period remains unknown. However, it is likely that most if not all of the measures undertaken by the senior author during revision TAR are performed by other foot and ankle surgeons during revision surgery regardless of prosthetic design or procedures performed. Future study regarding which, if any, of these measures are most effective and fiscally responsible should be undertaken.

In conclusion, the authors present a single surgeon's initial experience with revision of the Agility and Agility LP Total Ankle Replacement Systems through a case series of consecutive revisions to compare the safety of primary and revision TAR during the surgeon learning curve period as determined by the incidence of complications in the intraoperative and early postoperative period. When compared with the incidence of complications encountered for primary implantation of the Agility Total Ankle Replacement System encountered during the surgeon learning curve period, the results during a single surgeon's learning curve period for revision Agility and Agility Total Ankle Replacement Systems were highly favorable. Furthermore, they compared the incidence of low-grade complications as determined by the classification systems of Glazebrook and colleagues[16] and of Gadd and colleagues[17] and found revision Agility and Agility Total Ankle Replacement Systems to be safer than primary Agility and Agility Total Ankle Replacement when performed meticulously by a qualified foot and ankle surgeon during their learning curve period. A validated classification system for complications encountered during TAR regardless of prosthetic design is needed to allow for more standardized reporting of complications, irrespective of whether they are primary or revision TAR. Further still, more case series reporting on revision TAR complications during the initial learning surgeon learning curve period with separation of patient cohorts into early and late groups would then allow for systematic review and more homogenous analysis for a clinically significant incidence of complications during the revision TAR surgeon learning curve period.

REFERENCES

1. Clement RC, Krynetskiy E, Parekh SG. The total ankle arthroplasty learning curve with third-generation implants. Foot Ankle Spec 2013;6:263–70.
2. Saltzman CL, Mann RA, Ahrens JE, et al. Prospective controlled trial of STAR total ankle replacement versus ankle fusion: initial results. Foot Ankle Int 2009;30: 579–96.
3. Esparragoza L, Vidal C, Vaquero J. Comparative study of the quality of life between arthrodesis and total arthroplasty substitution of the ankle. J Foot Ankle Surg 2011;50:383–7.
4. Myerson MS, Mroczek K. Peri-operative complications of total ankle arthroplasty. Foot Ankle Int 2003;24:17–21.
5. Natens P, Dereymaeker G, Abbara M, et al. Early results after four years experience with the STAR uncemented total ankle prosthesis. Acta Orthop Belg 2003; 69:49–58.
6. Murnaghan JM, Warnock DS, Henderson SA. Total ankle replacement. Early experiences with STAR prosthesis. Ulster Med J 2005;74:9–13.
7. Schuberth JM, Patel S, Zarutsky E. Peri-operative complications of the Agility total ankle replacement in 50 initial, consecutive cases. J Foot Ankle Surg 2006;45: 139–46.
8. Kumar A, Dhar S. Total ankle replacement: early results during learning period. Foot Ankle Surg 2007;13:19–23.
9. Reuver JM, Dayerizadeh N, Burger B, et al. Total ankle replacement outcome in low volume centers: short-term follow-up. Foot Ankle Int 2010;31:1064–8.
10. Bleazey ST, Brigido SA, Protzman NM. Peri-operative complications of a modular stem fixed-bearing total ankle replacement with intramedullary guidance. J Foot Ankle Surg 2013;52:36–41.
11. Noelle S, Egidy CC, Cross MB, et al. Complication rates after total ankle arthroplasty in one hundred consecutive prostheses. Int Orthop 2013;37:1789–94.
12. Schimmel JJ, Walschot LH, Louwerens JW. Comparison of the short-term results of the first and last 50 Scandinavian Total Ankle Replacements: assessment of the learning curve in a consecutive series. Foot Ankle Int 2013;35:326–33.
13. Willegger M, Trnka HJ, Schuh R. The HINTEGRA ankle arthroplasty: intermediate term results of 16 consecutive ankles and a review on the current literature. Clin Res Foot Ankle 2013;2:124.

14. Saltzman CL, Amendola A, Anderson R, et al. Surgeon training and complications in total ankle arthroplasty. Foot Ankle Int 2003;24:514–8.
15. Criswell BJ, Douglas K, Naik R, et al. High revision and reoperation rates using the Agility total ankle system. Clin Orthop Relat Res 2012;470:1980–6.
16. Glazebrook MA, Arsenault K, Dunbar M. Evidence-based classification of complications in total ankle arthroplasty. Foot Ankle Int 2009;30:945–9.
17. Gadd RJ, Barwick TW, Paling E, et al. Assessment of a three-grade classification of complications in total ankle replacement. Foot Ankle Int 2014;35:434–7.
18. Gould JS. Revision total ankle arthroplasty. Am J Orthop 2005;34:361.
19. Raikin SM, Myerson MS. Avoiding and managing complications of the Agility total ankle replacement system. Orthop 2006;29:931–8.
20. Gupta S, Ellington JK, Myerson MS. Management of specific complications after revision total ankle replacement. Semin Arthroplasty 2010;21:310–9.
21. Jonck JH, Myerson MS. Revision total ankle replacement. Foot Ankle Clin N Am 2012;17:687–706.
22. McCollum G, Myerson MS. Failure of the Agility total ankle replacement system and salvage options. Clin Podiatr Med Surg 2013;30:207–23.
23. Besse JL, Beverhage BD, Leemrijse T. Revision total ankle replacements. Tech Foot Ankle Surg 2011;10:176–88.
24. Espinosa N, Wirth SH. Revision of the aseptic and septic total ankle replacement. Clin Podiatr Med Surg 2013;30:171–85.
25. Barg A, Horisberger M, Paul J, et al. Salvage procedures after failed total ankle replacement. Fuß Sprung 2013;11:228–37.
26. DeVries JG, Scott RT, Berlet GC, et al. Agility to INBONE: anterior and posterior approaches to the difficult revision total ankle replacement. Clin Podiatr Med Surg 2013;30:81–96.
27. Meeker J, Wegner N, Francisco R, et al. Revision techniques in total ankle arthroplasty using a stemmed tibial arthroplasty system. Tech Foot Ankle Surg 2013;12:99–108.
28. Penner MJ. Failed ankle replacement and conversion to arthrodesis: a treatment algorithm. Tec Foot Ankle 2012;11:125–32.
29. Donnenwerth M, Roukis TS. Tibio-talo-calcaneal arthrodesis with retrograde intramedullary compression nail fixation for salvage of failed total ankle replacement: a systematic review. Clin Podiatr Med Surg 2013;30:199–206.
30. DeOrio JK. Revision INBONE total ankle replacement. Clin Podiatr Med Surg 2013;30:225–36.
31. Horisberger M, Paul J, Wiewiorski M, et al. Commercially available trabecular metal ankle interpositional spacer for tibiotalocalcaneal arthrodesis secondary to severe bone loss of the ankle. J Foot Ankle Surg 2014;53:383–7.
32. Henricson A, Carlsson Å, Rydholm U. What is a revision of total ankle replacement? Foot Ankle Surg 2011;17:99–102.
33. Roukis TS. Incidence of revision after primary implantation of the agility total ankle replacement system: a systematic review. J Foot Ankle Surg 2012;51:198–204.
34. Roukis TS. Management of the failed Agility total ankle replacement system. Foot Ankle Q 2013;24:185–97.
35. Bestic JM, Bancroft LW, Peterson JJ, et al. Postoperative imaging of the total ankle arthroplasty. Radiol Clin North Am 2008;46:1003–15.
36. Roukis TS. Modified Evans peroneus brevis lateral ankle stabilization for balancing varus ankle contracture during total ankle replacement. J Foot Ankle Surg 2013;52:789–92.

37. Roukis TS, Prissel MA. Management of extensive tibial osteolysis with the Agility total ankle replacement systems using geometric metal-reinforced polymethyl-methacrylate cement augmentation. J Foot Ankle Surg 2014;53:101–7.

38. Roukis TS, Prissel MA. Management of extensive talar osteolysis with the Agility total ankle replacement systems using geometric metal-reinforced polymethyl-methacrylate cement augmentation. J Foot Ankle Surg 2014;53:108–13.

39. Roukis TS. Tibialis posterior recession for balancing varus ankle contracture during total ankle replacement. J Foot Ankle Surg 2013;52:686–9.

40. Roukis TS, Prissel MA. Reverse Evans peroneus brevis medial ankle stabilization for balancing valgus ankle contracture during total ankle replacement. J Foot Ankle Surg 2014;53:497–502.

41. Raikin SM. Avoiding wound complications in total ankle arthroplasty: surgical technique and tips. J Bone Joint Surg Essent Surg Tech 2011;1–A:e6.

42. Ellington JK, Gupta S, Myerson MS. Management of failures of total ankle replacement with the agility total ankle arthroplasty. J Bone Joint Surg 2013; 95–A:2112–8.

43. Roukis TS, Prissel MA. Revision of agility total ankle replacements using agility components is the right choice, sometimes. J Foot Ankle Surg 2014;53:391–3.

44. Roukis TS. Bacterial skin contamination prior to and after surgical preparation of the foot, ankle, and lower leg in patients with diabetes and intact skin versus patients with diabetes and ulceration: a prospective controlled therapeutic study. J Foot Ankle Surg 2010;49:348–56.

45. Schade VL, Roukis TS. Use of a surgical preparation and sterile dressing change during office visit treatment of chronic foot and ankle wounds decreases the incidence of infection and treatment costs. Foot Ankle Spec 2008;1:147–54.

46. Schweinberger MH, Roukis TS. Effectiveness of instituting a specific bed protocol n reducing complications associated with bed rest. J Foot Ankle Surg 2010;49: 340–7.

47. Abicht BP, Roukis TS. The INBONE II total ankle replacement system. Clin Podiatr Med Surg 2013;30:47–68.

48. Reilingh ML, Beimers L, Tuijthof GJ, et al. Measuring hindfoot alignment radiographically: the long axial view is more reliable than the hindfoot alignment view. Skel Radiol 2010;39:1103–8.

49. Available at: http://www.nzoa.org.nz/system/files/NZJR2014Report.pdf. Accessed July 18, 2015.

50. Schuberth JM, Steck JK, Christensen JC. Ill-conceived total ankle revision technique. J Foot Ankle Surg 2014;53:390–1.

51. Pyevich MT, Saltzman CL, Callaghan JJ, et al. Total ankle arthroplasty: a unique design. Two to twelve-year follow-up. J Bone Joint Surg 1998;80–A:1410–20.

52. Alvine FG. The Agility ankle replacement: the good and the bad. Foot Ankle Clin 2002;7:737–53.

53. Alvine FG. Design and development of the Agility ankle. Foot Ankle Spec 2009;2: 45–50.

54. Myerson MS, Won HY. Primary and revision total ankle replacement using custom-designed prosthesis. Foot Ankle Clin 2008;13:521–38.

55. Cerrato R, Myerson MS. Total ankle replacement: the Agility LP prosthesis. Foot Ankle Clin 2008;3:485–94.

56. Castro MD. Agility low profile: short-term update and representative case presentation. Sem Arthrop 2010;21:267–74.

57. Ketz J, Myerson M, Sanders R. The salvage of complex hindfoot problems with use of a custom talar total ankle prosthesis. J Bone Joint Surg 2012;94–A:1194–200.

58. Noriega F, Villanueva P, Moracia I, et al. Custom-made talar component in primary young patients and total ankle replacement revision: short-term results. J Bone Joint Surg 2011;93–B(Suppl II):148.

59. Roukis TS. Salvage of a failed DePuy Alvine total ankle prosthesis with agility LP custom stemmed tibia and talar components. Clin Podiatr Med Surg 2013;30: 101–9.

60. Myerson MS, Shariff R, Zonno AJ. The management of infection following total ankle replacement: demographics and treatment. Foot Ankle Int 2014;35(9): 855–62.

61. Schuberth JM, Christensen JC, Rialson JA. Metal-reinforced cement augmentation for complex talar subsidence in failed total ankle arthroplasty. J Foot Ankle Surg 2011;50:766–72.

62. Ferrao P, Myerson MS, Schuberth JM, et al. Cement spacer as definitive management for postoperative ankle infection. Foot Ankle Int 2012;33:173–8.

Management of Massive Hindfoot Osteolysis Secondary to Failed INBONE I Total Ankle Replacement

Thomas S. Roukis, DPM, PhD

KEYWORDS

- Arthroplasty • Complications • Fixed bearing polyethylene insert • Prosthesis
- Surgery

KEY POINTS

- Aseptic osteolysis, driven by phagocytosable polyethylene wear debris and initiated by macrophage activation, is the major cause of failure of total ankle replacement and results in loss of fixation of the prosthesis caused by osteoclast-mediated loss of bone.

- Bone loss presents a difficult problem for revision ankle replacement with limited options beyond impaction bone grafting, metal reinforced polymethyl methacrylate cement augmentation, or custom prosthesis. Bone grafting may be used to restore bone stock, and custom stemmed prosthesis and metal-reinforced cement may maximize fixation in cases with severe bone loss.

- Conversion of a failed INBONE I saddle talar component and polyethylene insert associated with massive aseptic osteolysis within the talus and calcaneus can be successfully treated with impaction cancellous allograft bone graft and conversion to an INBONE II sulcus talar component and polyethylene insert.

INTRODUCTION

The development of aseptic osteolysis following total ankle replacement is the major cause of failure, increases with time, and results in loss of fixation of the prosthesis. In brief, this process involves a macrophage-mediated osteolytic destruction of periprosthetic bone secondary to phagocytosable polyethylene wear debris usually as a result of component malposition.[1-11] Tibial and talar aseptic osteolysis either does or does not involve subsidence of the prosthetic components and component

Financial Disclosure: None reported.

Conflict of Interest: None reported.

Orthopaedic Center, Gundersen Health System, Mail Stop: CO2-006, 1900 South Avenue, La Crosse, WI 54601, USA

E-mail address: tsroukis@gundersenhealth.org

loosening may or may not exist. Regardless of the specific total ankle replacement system used, the bone loss associated with aseptic osteolysis can be quite extensive.[12–14]

The treatment of aseptic osteolysis during revision of the Agility Total Ankle Replacement Systems (DePuy Orthopaedics, Warsaw, IN)[5,13–23] and other total ankle replacement systems[2,3,24–29] has been described and predominantly involves curettage of the cystic cavities, impaction cancellous bone grafting or metal-reinforced polymethyl methacrylate cement augmentation, and component replacement. In reviewing the published literature involving the INBONE Total Ankle Replacement Systems (Wright Medical Technologies, Inc, Memphis, TN), the management of extensive aseptic osteolysis for these devices has not been reported.[24–26,30–35] The author presents a case of severe aseptic osteolysis of the talus and calcaneus along previous screw paths following triple arthrodesis and INBONE I Total Ankle Replacement (Wright Medical Technologies) that was successfully revised with curettage of the cystic cavity, impaction cancellous bone grafting supplemented with polymethyl methacrylate cement augmentation, and talar component replacement to the INBONE II Total Ankle Replacement (Wright Medical Technologies).

In September 1991 the patient was the passenger on a motorcycle and had her left foot/leg crushed between the bumper of a car and the motorcycle peg sustaining several puncture wounds about the posterior-lateral left lower leg/ankle. Below-knee amputation was recommended but refused by her brother who was the only family member that could be contacted at the time of her care. The foot injury was treated with pin fixation and thigh-high cast immobilization and she related being on antibiotics for an extended period of time but denied any severe infections developing, need for flaps, or skin grafting. As a result of persistent pain, the following year she underwent pin removal because of loosening and talonavicular arthrodesis left foot. She underwent several subsequent foot/ankle-related surgeries to resect osseous prominences and correct toe-related contractures. Progressive degenerative changes predominantly to the ankle joint and a lesser extent to the subtalar joint developed. In December 2007 she underwent subtalar and calcaneocuboid arthrodesis with takedown and repositional arthrodesis of the talonavicular joint thereby created a triple arthrodesis. An equinus contracture and progressive changes of her ankle joint ensued. At age 52 years, in January 2009, she underwent uncemented size 2 INBONE I Total Ankle Replacement with size 2, 8-mm polyethylene insert; internal fixation removal from the foot; and open posterior-central Strayer type gastrocnemius recession of the left lower leg. She was followed closely over the next 2 years by her primary podiatric provider with serial clinical examination and weight-bearing radiographs with intermittent computed tomography (CT) including three-dimensional reconstruction being obtained (**Figs. 1–4**). At the time of referral to the author, she was experiencing pain with activities globally about the anterior aspect of the ankle, medial gutter, and dorsal midfoot. She had noticed the ankle having less motion over time and also that she developed worsening toe-walking with external rotation of her foot. She is a self-described avid outdoors and exercise enthusiast enjoying bobsledding and wilderness camping; in April 2009 she developed an interest in triathlons to have a goal for her total ankle replacement rehabilitation.

Clinical examination revealed severely restricted sagittal plane range of motion with an osseous end-feel to dorsiflexion of the ankle. She had 0° of dorsiflexion and 10° of plantarflexion and the limited ankle motion was painful and had crepitus associated. No frontal plane ankle instability was appreciated. Pain to palpation of the entire anterior ankle joint line and to a lesser extent the medial gutter was appreciated. The previous incisions were all well healed and without hypertrophy or tethering to the

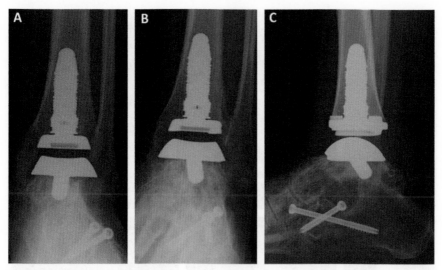

Fig. 1. Weight bearing anterior-posterior (*A*), oblique (*B*), and lateral (*C*) ankle radiographs obtained in November 2011, 22 months following primary insertion of an INBONE I Total Ankle Replacement System. Common to the INBONE I Total Ankle Replacement System, the talar component is oversized relative to the native talar body width. Note that the previously performed triple arthrodesis is mature, hardware about the talonavicular and subtalar joint arthrodesis sites has been removed, and cystic changes about the talar neck and calcaneal body are appreciated.

underlying tissues. There were no cardinal signs of infection appreciated and she had intact epicritic sensation throughout her foot, ankle, and lower leg. Doppler examination revealed audible anterior tibial, perforating peroneal, and posterior tibial arteries with intact communication through the first perforating artery in the first webspace. Weight bearing and charger posture simulation revealed no meaningful dorsiflexion of the foot at the ankle. She walked with a limp, toe-walking when barefoot with the foot externally rotated, and had an early heel-off to the left side.

Radiographic studies (see **Figs. 1** and **3**) including multiple weight-bearing views of the left foot and ankle revealed 1° plantarflexion alignment between components (apex posterior) on the lateral view. Stress images revealed 0° dorsiflexion and 10° of plantarflexion relative to the resting component alignment and 1° heel varus. No evidence of tibial component migration or stress shielding with good coverage of the distal tibia was appreciated. The talar component was large, impinged on the medial and lateral malleoli, and appeared worsened since prior radiographs at the time of primary total ankle replacement. A sclerotic line beneath the talar component consistent with aseptic loosening was evident. Extensive cystic changes were appreciated in the talar neck and body and throughout the body of the calcaneus that appeared to have rapidly progressed since prior radiographs and had developed some enhanced trabecular bone about the talar component stem indicating stress-shielding.

The CT images including three-dimensional reconstructions (see **Figs. 2** and **4**) revealed a stable tibial component and no evidence of a fractured polyethylene insert. Extensive medial and lateral gutter impingement and degeneration was appreciated that had clearly worsened since the prior CT imaging. Despite the metallic artifact, the talar component demonstrated osteolysis anteriorly, medially, and laterally. Massive cystic changes are appreciated in the talar neck and body and throughout

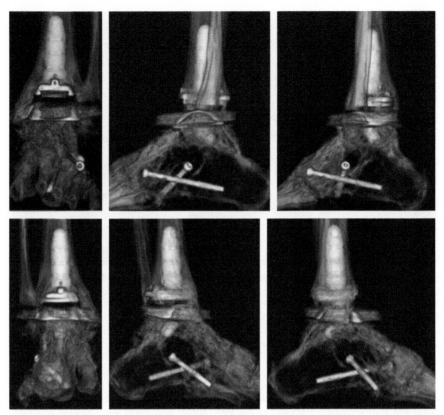

Fig. 2. Multiple computed tomography three-dimensional reconstruction images obtained at the same time as those demonstrated in **Fig. 1.** Note the obvious cystic changes throughout the talar neck and calcaneal body that are much more extensive than appreciated on the plain film radiographs.

the body of the calcaneus that had worsened since prior CT imaging and had enhanced trabecular bone about the talar component stem. Some of the cystic changes were obviously about the screw path for the subtalar fusion but even this had enlarged.

Having developed extensive and radiographically enlarging cystic changes within the entire remaining talus and calcaneus over a short period of time, the patient was counseled on operative intervention to limit the potential for catastrophic failure. Because custom stemmed or augmented talar components are not readily available in the United States,[15,17] the surgical choices were described as either a tibiotalocalcaneal arthrodesis using bulk femoral head allograft[36] and retrograde locked intramedullary nail stabilization or revision total ankle replacement with a sulcus talar component and polyethylene insert from the INBONE II Total Ankle Replacement System to replace her current saddle-shaped talar component and polyethylene insert. With either procedure, the cystic lesions within the talus and calcaneus would be resected and cancellous allograft impregnated with bone marrow aspirate from her ipsilateral proximal tibia[37] would be impaction grafted into the osseous defect. In addition, if total ankle replacement revision was performed the new talar component would be supported anteriorly with a mantle of polymethyl methacrylate cement with or without metal reinforcement[12–14] and a percutaneous tendo-Achilles lengthening[38] and

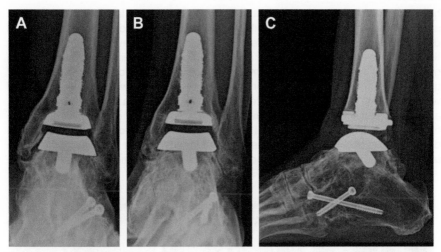

Fig. 3. Weight bearing anterior-posterior (*A*), oblique (*B*), and lateral (*C*) ankle radiographs obtained in October 2012, 33 months following primary insertion of an INBONE I Total Ankle Replacement System. Note the progressive medial and lateral gutter narrowing and spur formation along with osteolysis about the talar component. Note that the cystic changes about the talar neck and calcaneal body have progressed significantly since the previous radiographs obtained 11 months prior.

posterior capsule resection would be performed to enhance ankle joint dorsiflexion. The patient declined an arthrodesis as a first-line treatment option but agreed to the revision total ankle replacement.

SURGICAL TECHNIQUE

Under general anesthesia with a left-sided femoral and popliteal indwelling catheter nerve blockade, her previous anterior ankle incision was used overlying the extensor

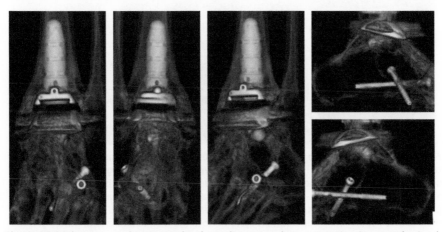

Fig. 4. Multiple computed tomography three-dimensional reconstruction images obtained at the same time as those demonstrated in **Fig. 3**. Note the markedly worsened cystic changes throughout the entire talar head/neck and calcaneal body with the only appreciable bone supporting the talar stem.

hallucis longus tendon and the junction between this tendon laterally and the tibialis anterior tendon maintained within its sheath medially was developed and carried down to the underlying ankle joint. Next the periosteum was elevated off of the anterior tibia and talus and exposed the prior ankle joint replacement that revealed subsidence of the anterior aspect of the talar component as expected clinically (**Fig. 5**A). The scar tissue about the prosthetic components and polyethylene wear debris embedded within the ankle capsule were resected to expose the full width of the medial, anterior, and lateral joint line. The polyethylene insert was fenestrated, disarticulated from the tibial tray, and removed. The tibial tray was deemed sound and left in situ. The dome of the talar component was then removed from the stem by releasing the Morse taper. The medial and lateral gutters of the malleoli and talar/calcaneal side-walls were

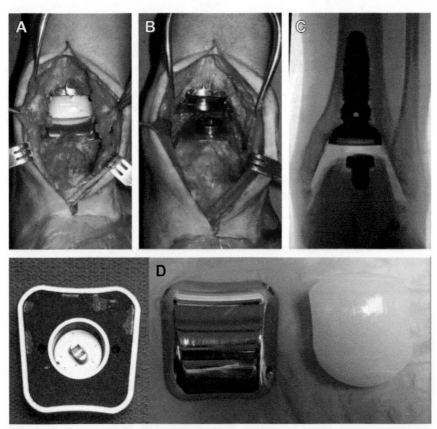

Fig. 5. Intraoperative photograph in December 2012 demonstrating subsidence of the talar component of the INBONE I Total Ankle Replacement System, impingement of the medial and lateral gutters, and extensive polyethylene debris imbedded within the periprosthetic ankle capsule (held in pick-up forceps) (A). Intraoperative photograph (B) and anterior-posterior image intensification view (C) after removal of the failed talar component of the INBONE I Total Ankle Replacement System. Note the medial and lateral gutter debridement, and metallic debris imbedded in the talar dome secondary to motion between the talar cap and stem. Intraoperative photographs, from left to right, of the inferior surface of the talar component revealing limited osseous on-growth, abrasion of the superior surface, and wear of the polyethylene insert (D).

carefully débrided to provide spacing and resolve impingement (see **Fig. 5**B, C). The posterior ankle capsule and ectopic bone was resected throughout to reduce the posterior restraint. Inspection revealed poor osseous on-growth with subsidence consistent with the preoperative imaging studies (see **Fig. 5**D). The contents of the hindfoot fusion mass about the talus and calcaneus was then resected with hand instrumentation and revealed a massive osseous defect consistent with the preoperative imaging studies (**Fig. 6**). Next the osseous defect was packed with 60 mL of cancellous bone

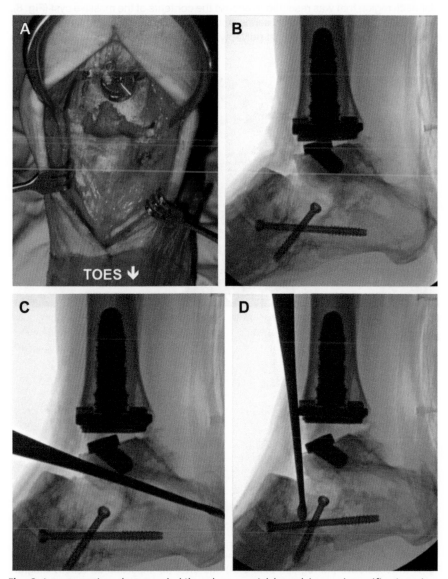

Fig. 6. Intraoperative photograph (A) and sequential lateral image intensification views (B–D) demonstrating the massive osseous defect within the talar head/neck and calcaneus following curettage and evacuation of the cystic contents. Note the preservation of the talar stem within the posterior aspect of the talar body.

allograft mixed with bone marrow aspirate harvested from her proximal tibia. The mixture was impaction grafted into the osseous defect (**Fig. 7**). Next the trial talar component was placed and determined to be a size 2 sulcus with an 8-mm size 2 polyethylene insert. Despite resection of the posterior ankle capsule and through medial and lateral gutter débridement, ankle joint dorsiflexion was limited and a percutaneous tendo-Achilles lengthening performed to achieve 10° of dorsiflexion intraoperatively. The trial components were removed and the definitive talar dome secured to the talar stem with antibiotic-impregnated polymethyl methacrylate cement about the anterior talar neck region that was resected to access the contents of the massive cyst (**Fig. 8**). This was verified with anterior-posterior, oblique, and lateral intraoperative C-arm image intensification views. The final polyethylene insert was then placed securely into

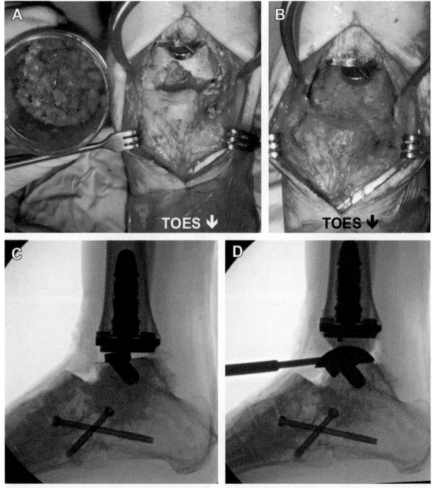

Fig. 7. Intraoperative photograph before (*A*) and after (*B*) impaction cancellous allograft bone grafting impregnated with bone marrow aspirate concentrate harvested from the ipsilateral proximal tibia. Lateral image intensification view following impaction cancellous allograft bone grafting (*C*). Lateral image intensification view following coupling of the revision talar component from the INBONE II Total Ankle Replacement System (*D*).

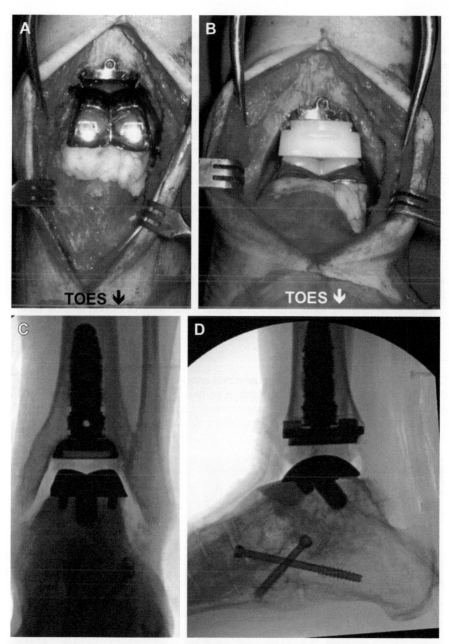

Fig. 8. Intraoperative photograph before (*A*) and after insertion of the polyethylene insert (*B*) following application of polymethyl methacrylate cement to support the anterior aspect of the talar component and fill the anterior talar neck osseous defect. Anterior-posterior (*C*) and lateral (*D*) image intensification demonstrating good medial and lateral gutter space following débridement, and filled osseous cystic defect with impaction cancellous allograft bone grafting and polymethyl methacrylate cement supporting the anterior aspect of the INBONE II Total Ankle Replacement System talar component.

the joint space and impacted until fully engaged. The ankle was then placed through full range of motion and revealed appropriate range of motion and stability against anterior-posterior and inversion-eversion displacement. This was verified with anterior-posterior and lateral intraoperative C-arm image intensification stress views.

Throughout the procedure the surgical site was irrigated with copious amounts of sterile saline impregnated with antibiotic using a power lavage system. The surgical site was closed in layers over a suction drain and initially stabilized with a plaster splint. On the third postoperative day the drain was removed and a short leg fiberglass cast applied with the foot held in neutral alignment relative to the lower leg.

She healed her incision primarily and, after remaining strict non–weight bearing for 12 weeks, enrolled in a structured physical therapy program to restore dorsiflexion motion and plantarflexion power, release scar tissue about the anterior ankle incision that was tethering the underlying extensor hallucis longus tendon, and gradually return to nonballistic physical activities over an additional 6 months.

CLINICAL OUTCOME

Except for some expected rebound peripheral edema, no untoward complications occurred and the patient progressed to return of full ambulation and nonimpact exercise. At 3-year follow-up, the patient has a well aligned, stable, and pain-free total ankle replacement with functional sagittal plane ankle range of motion to allow for unimpeded gait (**Fig. 9**).

COMPLICATIONS AND CONCERNS

The patient continues to undergo routine oral antibiotic prophylaxis for dental procedures. Additionally, she avoids ambulation on uneven ground and ballistic activities. Although in the laboratory setting the sulcus talar component and polyethylene design of the INBONE II Total Ankle Replacement System has been demonstrated to

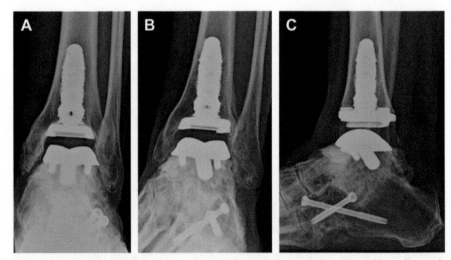

Fig. 9. Anterior-posterior (A), oblique (B), and lateral (C) weight bearing ankle radiographs obtained 3 years following revision demonstrating full osseous incorporation of the impaction cancellous bone grafting and stable polymethyl methacrylate cement and talar component alignment.

experience less stress than the saddle talar component and polyethylene design of the INBONE II Total Ankle Replacement System, it remains to be seen if this correlates with less polyethylene debris wear and aseptic osteolysis. It will be necessary to monitor her long-term for potential talar component subsidence because of the previous massive aseptic osteolysis and because polymethyl methacrylate cement was used to affix the anterior talar component. Conversion to a tibiotalocalcaneal arthrodesis would be challenging and require use of a bulk femoral head or tibial allograft[36,39] or metallic interpositional spacer[40,41] with the known risks associated with these forms of limb salvage. The use of a fixed ankle-foot orthosis remains plausible if she develops symptoms that warrant this form of functional bracing.

Perhaps in the future if a similar clinical scenario (previous triple arthrodesis undergoing a primary total ankle replacement) presented, the screw paths within bone about the hindfoot and midfoot could be impaction bone grafted immediately following removal. This may reduce the pathway for polyethylene wear debris to enter into these defects and accordingly the development of aseptic osteolysis.[2,4] Additionally, the effect on outcome of US Food and Drug Administration clearance of total ankle replacement with polymethyl methacrylate that are instead implanted without cement, as occurred with the case presented here, remains unanswered.[12,18]

SUMMARY

This article presents a procedure whereby a failed INBONE I saddle talar component and polyethylene insert associated with massive cystic changes within the talus and calcaneus secondary to aseptic osteolysis was treated with impaction cancellous allograft bone graft impregnated with autogenous proximal tibia bone marrow aspirate and conversion to an INBONE II sulcus talar component and polyethylene insert. A percutaneous tendo-Achilles lengthening and posterior capsule release was performed to enhance ankle dorsiflexion. In context, the rationale for these procedures, operative sequence of events, and recovery course are presented in detail. Causes for concern regarding subsequent revision should this be required were raised.

REFERENCES

1. Assal M, Al-Shaikh R, Reiber BH, et al. Fracture of the polyethylene component in an ankle arthroplasty: a case report. Foot Ankle Int 2003;24:901–3.
2. Espinosa N, Wirth SH. Revision of the aseptic and septic total ankle replacement. Clin Podiatr Med Surg 2013;30:171–85.
3. Fukuda T, Haddad SL, Ren Y, et al. Impact of talar component rotation on contact pressure after total ankle arthroplasty: a cadaveric study. Foot Ankle Int 2010;31:404–11.
4. Gaden MTR, Ollivere BJ. Periprosthetic aseptic osteolysis in total ankle replacement: cause and management. Clin Podiatr Med Surg 2013;30:145–55.
5. Hanna RS, Haddad SL, Lazarus ML. Evaluation of periprosthetic lucency after total ankle arthroplasty: helical CT versus conventional radiography. Foot Ankle Int 2007;28:921–6.
6. Ingham E, Fisher J. Biological reactions to wear debris in total joint replacement. Proc Inst Mech Eng H 2000;214:21–37.
7. Kohonen I, Koivu H, Pudas T, et al. Does computed tomography add information on radiographic analysis in detecting periprosthetic osteolysis after total ankle arthroplasty? Foot Ankle Int 2013;34:180–8.
8. Kobayashi A, Minoda Y, Kadoya Y, et al. Ankle arthroplasties generate wear particles similar to knee arthroplasties. Clin Orthop Relat Res 2004;(424):69–72.

9. Nicholson JJ, Parks BG, Stroud C, et al. Joint contact characteristics in Agility total ankle arthroplasty. Clin Orthop Rel Res 2004;(424):125–9.

10. Van Boerum DH, Morgan JM, Dockter ER. Periprosthetic fractures: intraoperative and postoperative. Chapter 17. In: Coetzee JC, Hurwitz SR, editors. Arthritis & arthroplasty: the foot and ankle. Philadelphia: Saunders Elsevier; 2010. p. 146–52.

11. Vaupel Z, Baker EA, Baker KC, et al. Analysis of retrieved Agility™ total ankle arthroplasty systems. Foot Ankle Int 2009;30:815–23.

12. Roukis TS. Management of the failed Agility™ total ankle replacement system. Foot Ankle Quarterly 2013;24:185–97.

13. Prissel MA, Roukis TS. Management of extensive tibial osteolysis with the Agility™ total ankle replacement systems using geometric metal-reinforced polymethylmethacrylate cement augmentation. J Foot Ankle Surg 2014;53:101–7.

14. Roukis TS, Prissel MA. Management of extensive talar osteolysis with the Agility™ total ankle replacement systems using geometric metal-reinforced polymethylmethacrylate cement augmentation. J Foot Ankle Surg 2014;53:108–13.

15. Ketz J, Myerson M, Sanders R. The salvage of complex hindfoot problems with use of a custom talar total ankle prosthesis. J Bone Joint Surg Am 2012;94: 1194–200.

16. McCollum G, Myerson MS. Failure of the Agility™ total ankle replacement system and the salvage options. Clin Podiatr Med Surg 2013;30:207–23.

17. Roukis TS. Salvage of a failed "DePuy Alvine Total Ankle Prosthesis" with Agility™ LP custom stemmed tibial and talar components. Clin Podiatr Med Surg 2013;30: 101–9.

18. Roukis TS. Incidence of revision after primary implantation of the Agility™ total ankle replacement system: a systematic review. J Foot Ankle Surg 2012;51: 198–204.

19. Haddad SL. Revision Agility total ankle arthroplasty. Chapter 76. In: Easley ME, Wiesel SW, editors. Operative techniques in foot and ankle surgery. Philadelphia: Lippincott Williams & Wilkins; 2011. p. 622–42.

20. Jonck JH, Myerson MS. Revision total ankle replacement. Foot Ankle Clin 2012; 17:687–706.

21. Myerson MS. Revision total ankle replacement. Chapter 25. In: Myerson MS, editor. Reconstructive foot and ankle surgery: management of complications. 2nd edition. Philadelphia: Elsevier Saunders; 2010. p. 295–316.

22. Sanders RW. Failed total ankle arthroplasty. Chapter 30. In: Nunley JA, Pfeffer GB, Sanders RW, et al, editors. Advanced reconstruction: foot and ankle. Rosemont (IL): American Academy of Orthopaedic Surgeons; 2004. p. 201–8.

23. Sanders R. Recognition and salvage of the failed ankle replacement arthroplasty. Chapter 20. In: Coetzee JC, Hurwitz SR, editors. Arthritis & arthroplasty: the foot and ankle. Philadelphia: Saunders Elsevier; 2010. p. 178–86.

24. Meeker J, Wegner N, Francisco R, et al. Revision techniques in total ankle arthroplasty utilizing a stemmed tibial arthroplasty system. Tech Foot Ankle Surg 2013; 12:99–108.

25. Schuberth JM, Christensen JC, Rialson JA. Metal-reinforced cement augmentation for complex talar subsidence in failed total ankle arthroplasty. J Foot Ankle Surg 2011;50:766–72.

26. DeOrio JK. Revision INBONE total ankle replacement. Clin Podiatr Med Surg 2013;30:225–36.

27. Prissel M, Roukis TS. Incidence of revision following primary insertion of the STAR™ implant: a systematic review. Clin Podiatr Med Surg 2013;30:237–50.

28. Hintermann B. Complications of total ankle arthroplasty. Chapter 11. In: Hintermann B, editor. Total ankle arthroplasty: historical overview, current concepts, and future perspectives. New York: Springer; 2005. p. 163–84.
29. Hintermann B. Salvage of failed total ankle arthroplasty, Procedure 26. In: Pfeffer GB, Easley ME, Frey C, et al, editors. Operative techniques: foot and ankle surgery. Philadelphia: Saunders; 2010. p. 325–40.
30. DeOrio JK. Focus on total ankle arthroplasty. Orthopedics 2006;29:978–80.
31. Reiley MA. INBONE™ total ankle replacement. Foot Ankle Spec 2008;1:118–22.
32. Ellis S, DeOrio JK. The INBONE™ total ankle replacement. Oper Tech Orthop 2010;20:201–10.
33. DeOrio JK. Total ankle replacement with subtalar arthrodesis. Management of combined ankle and subtalar arthritis. Tech Foot Ankle Surg 2010;9:182–9.
34. Abicht BP, Roukis TS. The INBONE™ II total ankle replacement system. Clin Podiatr Med Surg 2013;30:47–68.
35. Bleazey ST, Brigido SA, Protzman NM. Perioperative complications of a modular stem fixed-bearing total ankle replacement with intramedullary guidance. J Foot Ankle Surg 2013;52:36–41.
36. Donnenwerth M, Roukis TS. Tibio-talo-calcaneal arthrodesis with retrograde intramedullary compression nail fixation for salvage of failed total ankle replacement: a systematic review. Clin Podiatr Med Surg 2013;30:199–206.
37. Schweinberger MH, Roukis TS. Percutaneous autologous bone-marrow harvest from the calcaneus and proximal tibia: surgical technique. J Foot Ankle Surg 2007;46:411–4.
38. Schweinberger MH, Roukis TS. Surgical correction of soft-tissue ankle equinus contracture. Clin Podiatr Med Surg 2008;25:571–85.
39. Penner MJ. Failed ankle replacement and conversion to arthrodesis: a treatment algorithm. Tech Foot Ankle Surg 2012;11:125–32.
40. Henricson A, Rydholm U. Use of a trabecular metal implant in ankle arthrodesis after failed total ankle replacement. Acta Orthop 2010;81:745–7.
41. Horisberger M, Paul J, Wiewiorski M, et al. Commercially available trabecular metal ankle interpositional spacer for tibiotalocalcaneal arthrodesis secondary to severe bone loss of the ankle. J Foot Ankle Surg 2014;53:383–7.

Salvage of a Failed Agility Total Ankle Replacement System Associated with Acute Traumatic Periprosthetic Midfoot Fractures

(R) CrossMark

Thomas S. Roukis, DPM, PhD

KEYWORDS

- Arthroplasty • Complications • Fixed bearing polyethylene insert • Prosthesis
- Surgery

KEY POINTS

- Strategies for periprosthetic fracture management involve anatomic reduction and stabilization of the prosthesis.
- Although commonly reported for the hip and knee, limited information is available regarding the management of periprosthetic fractures associated with total ankle replacement.
- Salvage of a failed total ankle replacement system through revision with simultaneous repair of periprosthetic midfoot fractures has not been previously reported.

INTRODUCTION

Periprosthetic fracture patterns and associated strategies for osteosynthesis following total hip and knee replacement[1-3] are well documented. More recently, individual case reports and small case series, as well as expert opinion literature have been published regarding the management of periprosthetic fractures associated with total ankle replacement.[4-9] While revision of the Agility Total Ankle Replacement Systems (DePuy Orthopaedics, Warsaw, Indiana) has been extensively reported,[10-23] to the author's knowledge, the simultaneous performance of revision total ankle replacement and

Financial Disclosure: None reported.
Conflict of Interest: None reported.
Orthopaedic Center, Gundersen Health System, Mail Stop: CO2-006, 1900 South Avenue, La Crosse, WI 54601, USA
E-mail address: tsroukis@gundersenhealth.org

concomitant osteosynthesis of periprosthetic fractures had not been previously reported. In this article, the author presents a rare case requiring simultaneous revision of a failed Agility Total Ankle Replacement System and open reduction with internal fixation of periprosthetic midfoot fractures.

In 1972, the patient sustained a closed left-sided pronation-external rotation ankle fracture–dislocation treated with open reduction and internal fixation. She healed her fractures but developed post-traumatic degenerative joint disease of the ankle associated with distal lateral tibia osteonecrosis. In March 2004, at age 60-years, she underwent an Agility Total Ankle Replacement with a size 3 tibial component, size 3 posterior augmented talar component, and bottom-loaded full-column neutral ultra-high molecular weight polyethylene (UHMWPE) insert. She had intermittent follow-up over the next 8-years. The author evaluated her in 2012 as part of a total ankle replacement surveillance program, during which radiographic surveillance revealed progressive posterior and lateral subsidence of the talar component, as well as extensive talar osteolysis (**Fig. 1**). Despite these findings, she remained pleased with her function, had no pain, and although the potential for revision total ankle replacement in the future was discussed, she declined this option and elected to continue with yearly surveillance. Unfortunately, shortly after her index visit with the author, she fell down a flight of stairs after being chased by a bat and sustained comminuted navicular and cuboid fractures, intercuneiform separation, and acute loosening of the talar component (**Fig. 2**). Computed tomography imaging confirmed the radiographic findings and also demonstrated extensive cystic changes within the talar head and neck adjacent to the subsided talar component (**Fig. 3**).

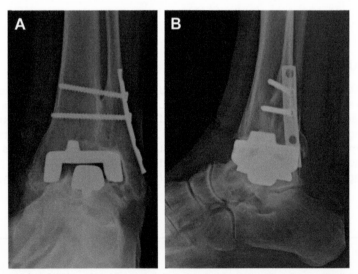

Fig. 1. Weight-bearing anterior–posterior (A) and lateral (B) ankle radiographs obtained 8 years following Agility Total Ankle Replacement with a posterior augmented talar component and fibular side plate and compression screw construct for distal tibio-fibular arthrodesis. Note the extensive cystic changes in the talar head–neck and severe talar component subsidence with varus and posterior angulation, as well as contact of the talar component fin with the subchondral bone about the subtalar joint.

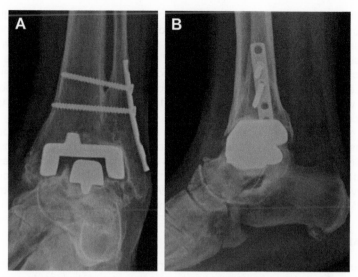

Fig. 2. Nonweight-bearing anterior–posterior (A) and lateral (B) ankle radiographs demonstrating loosening of the talar component, further subsidence, and fracture of the navicular and cuboid. Not shown in these images is diastasis between the cuneiforms.

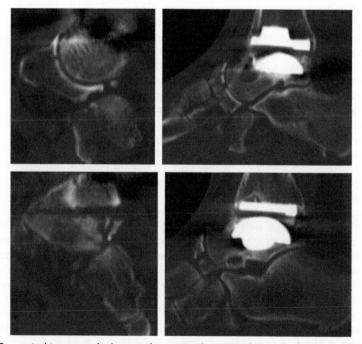

Fig. 3. Computed tomography images demonstrating extensive cystic changes within the talar head–neck region, degree of talar component subsidence, and displaced, comminuted fractures of the navicular and cuboid. Not shown in these images is diastasis between the cuneiforms.

Clinical examination revealed severely restricted sagittal plane range of motion with an osseous end-feel to dorsiflexion and limited plantarflexion of the ankle. The previous incisions were all well healed and without hypertrophy or tethering to the underlying tissues. There were no cardinal signs of infection appreciated, and the patient had intact epicritic sensation throughout her foot, ankle, and lower leg. Doppler examination revealed audible anterior tibial, perforating peroneal, and posterior tibial arteries with intact communication through the first perforating artery in the first webspace.

Open reduction with internal fixation of the extensive periprosthetic midfoot fractures was recommended to the patient. Additionally, based on pattern of subsidence and acute loosening of the talar component, as well as extensive cystic changes within the head and neck of the talus and the proximity to the periprosthetic midfoot fractures, revision of the talar component and UHMWPE insert with polymethylmethacrylate (PMMA) cement augmentation was recommended.

SURGICAL TECHNIQUE

Under general anesthesia with a left sided popliteal and saphenous nerve blockade, an anterior ankle incision was employed overlying the extensor halluces longus tendon and the junction between this tendon laterally and the anterior tibialis tendon medially. This interval was developed and carried down to the underlying tibia and talus. Resection of scar tissue, inflamed synovium, and soft tissues consistent with polyethylene wear debris allowed visualization of the prosthesis. The posterior augmented talar component was noted to be severely subsided into the talus as expected from the preoperative radiographic studies performed (**Fig. 4**). The UHMWPE insert was removed and revealed a deep groove consistent with asymmetric edge loading. The cystic changes were evacuated via curettage and the medial and lateral aspects of the talus contoured to relieve osseous impingement. Following irrigation with copious amounts of sterile saline impregnated with antibiotic using a power lavage system, PMMA cement augmentation of the cystic cavities was performed, and conversion to a size 3 revision talar component affixed to the talus with PMMA cement was performed (see **Fig. 4**). A bottom-loaded half column neutral UHMWPE insert was employed. It should be noted that the size 3 revision talar component added 2.1 mm of height relative to the size 3 posterior augmented talar component and allowed for proper tensioning of the ankle joint ligament complexes in this patient. Next, the anterior incision was extended distally and a separate incision employed over the cuboid to address the periprosthetic fractures treated with open reduction and internal fixation (**Fig. 5**).

Throughout the procedure the surgical site was irrigated with copious amounts of sterile saline impregnated with antibiotic using a power lavage system. The surgical site was closed in layers over a suction drain and initially stabilized with a plaster splint. On the third postoperative day, the drain was removed and a short leg fiberglass cast applied with the foot held in neutral alignment relative to the lower leg. Some superficial, noninfected necrosis of the lateral incision to treat the cuboid fracture developed that resolved with local wound care measures by postoperative week 8. Serial dressing and cast changes occurred over the first 8 postoperative weeks until radiographs confirmed osseous union of the patient's periprosthetic fractures. This was followed by use of a removable pneumatic-controlled ankle motion boot for an additional 4 weeks. The patient initiated full weight bearing at 8 weeks, was weaned out of the pneumatic boot into supportive shoe gear over the ensuing 4 weeks time, and gradually returned to her desired activities of daily living over the next 4 weeks.

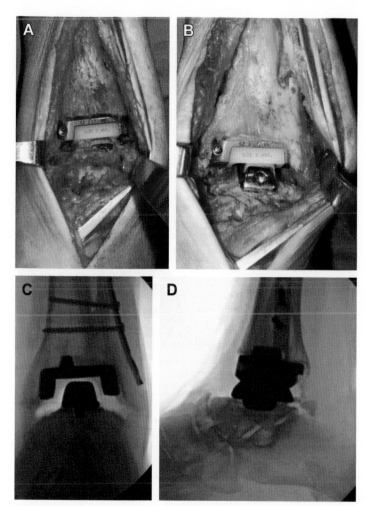

Fig. 4. Intraoperative photograph demonstrating subsidence and varus angulation of the posterior augmented talar component (*A*). Intraoperative photograph following PMMA cement augmentation of the revision talar component, bottom-loaded full column neutral UHMWPE insert and filling the cystic osseous defect within the talus with PMMA cement (*B*). Anterior–posterior (*C*) and lateral (*D*) intra-operative image intensification views demonstrating well-aligned revision talar component with neutral frontal and sagittal plane alignment. Note the extensive medial and lateral gutter débridement and PMMA cement mantle under the talar component and within the cysts.

CLINICAL OUTCOME

Except for some expected rebound peripheral edema, no further untoward complications occurred and the patient progressed to return of full ambulation and nonimpact exercise. At 2.5-year follow-up, the patient has a well-aligned, stable, and pain-free total ankle replacement with functional sagittal plane ankle range of motion to allow for unimpeded gait with no internal fixation related problems encountered **(Fig. 6)**.

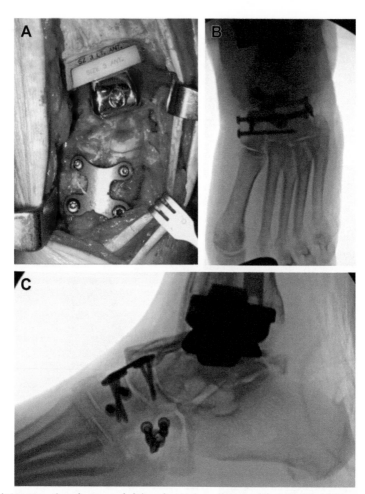

Fig. 5. Intraoperative photograph (*A*) and anterior–posterior (*B*) and lateral (*C*) image intensification views following open reduction of the comminuted navicular fracture using bridge plate and locking screw stabilization, intercuneiform joint stabilization and cuboid stabilization with cannulated compression screw fixation. Note the anatomic reduction of the fractures.

COMPLICATIONS AND CONCERNS

The lateral incision wound healing problem was attributed to the additional soft tissue dissection required to expose the cuboid adequately to perform the open reduction with internal fixation. However, it seems unlikely that healing the patient's wound primarily would have decreased the duration of immobilization or improved her early outcome.

The patient continues to undergo routine oral antibiotic prophylaxis for dental procedures. Additionally, she avoids ambulation on uneven ground and ballistic activities including extensive ambulation. It will be necessary to monitor her long-term for potential recurrent osteolysis and subsequent talar component subsidence due to the fact that polymethylmethacrylate cement was used to affix the talar component.

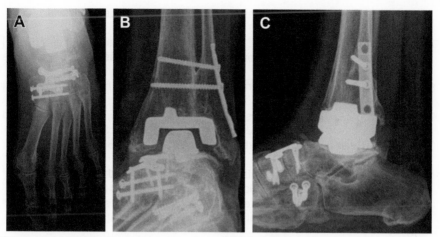

Fig. 6. Anterior–posterior (*A*), lateral dorsiflexion (*B*), and lateral plantarflexion (*C*) views obtained 2.5 years following revision of the Agility Total Ankle Replacement System and open reduction with internal fixation of the midfoot fractures. Note the full sagittal plane motion achieved, as well as maintained frontal and sagittal plane alignment and stability of the revision talar component.

Additionally, the development of subtalar joint degenerative joint disease requiring arthrodesis would be problematic to perform due to the limited bone stock that would remain, and conversion to a tibio-talo-calcaneal arthrodesis would be challenging and require use of a bulk femoral head or tibial allograft[8,9,24,25] or metallic interpositional spacer[26,27] with the known risks associated with these forms of limb salvage.

SUMMARY

The author presented a rare case involving combined revision of a failed Agility Total Ankle Replacement System and open reduction with internal fixation of periprosthetic midfoot fractures. In context, the rationale for these procedures, the operative sequence of events, and recovery course were presented in detail. Causes for concern regarding subsequent revision should this be required were raised.

REFERENCES

1. Pospula W, Abu Noor T. Periprosthetic fractures of the femur after hip and knee replacement. Med Princ Pract 2009;18:198–203.
2. Holzapel BM, Prodinger PM, Hoberg M, et al. Periprosthetic fractures after total hip arthroplasty: classification, diagnosis, and therapy strategies. Orthopade 2010;39:519–35 [in German].
3. Ochs BG, Stöckle U, Gebhard F. Interprosthetic fractures-a challenge of treatment. Eur Orthop Traumatol 2013;4:103–9.
4. Manegold S, Haas NP, Tsitsilonis S, et al. Periprosthetic fractures in total ankle replacement: classification system and treatment algorithm. J Bone Joint Surg Am 2013;95:815–20.
5. Castro MD. Insufficiency fractures after total ankle replacement. Tech Foot Ankle Surg 2007;6:15–21.
6. Van Boerum DH, Morgan JM, Dockter ER. Periprosthetic fractures: intraoperative and postoperative. Chapter 17. In: Coetzee JC, Hurwitz SR, editors. Arthritis &

arthroplasty: the foot and ankle. Philadelphia: Saunders Elsevier; 2010. p. 146–52.

7. Yang JH, Kim HJ, Yoon JR, et al. Minimally invasive plate osteosynthesis (MIPO) for periprosthetic fracture after total ankle arthroplasty: a case report. Foot Ankle Int 2011;32:200–4.

8. Penner MJ. Failed ankle replacement and conversion to arthrodesis: a treatment algorithm. Tech Foot Ankle Surg 2012;11:125–32.

9. DiDomenico LA, Thomas ZM. Use of femoral locking plate for salvage of failed ankle arthroplasty after trauma. J Foot Ankle Surg 2013;52:397–401.

10. Gould JS. Revision total ankle arthroplasty. Am J Orthop (Belle Mead NJ) 2005; 34:361.

11. Roukis TS. Incidence of revision after primary implantation of the Agility™ total ankle replacement system: a systematic review. J Foot Ankle Surg 2012;51:198–204.

12. Roukis TS. Salvage of a failed "DePuy Alvine Total Ankle Prosthesis" with Agility™ LP custom stemmed tibial and talar components. Clin Podiatr Med Surg 2013;30: 101–9.

13. Roukis TS. Management of the failed Agility™ total ankle replacement system. Foot Ankle Quarterly 2013;24:185–97.

14. Prissel MA, Roukis TS. Management of extensive tibial osteolysis with the Agility™ total ankle replacement systems using geometric metal-reinforced polymethyl-methacrylate cement augmentation. J Foot Ankle Surg 2014;53:101–7.

15. Roukis TS, Prissel MA. Management of extensive talar osteolysis with the Agility™ total ankle replacement systems using geometric metal-reinforced polymethyl-methacrylate cement augmentation. J Foot Ankle Surg 2014;53:108–13.

16. Roukis TS, Prissel MA. A closer look at total ankle revision. Podiatry Today 2014; 27:52–63.

17. Alvine FG. Total ankle arthroplasty: new concepts and approach. Contemp Orthop 1991;22:397–403.

18. Alvine FG. The Agility™ ankle replacement: the good and the bad. Foot Ankle Clin 2002;7:737–53.

19. Myerson MS. Revision total ankle replacement. Chapter 25. In: Myerson MS, editor. Reconstructive foot and ankle surgery: management of complications. 2nd edition. Philadelphia: Elsevier Saunders; 2010. p. 295–316.

20. Gupta S, Ellington JK, Myerson MS. Management of specific complications after revision total ankle replacement. Semin Arthroplasty 2010;21:310–9.

21. Jonck JH, Myerson MS. Revision total ankle replacement. Foot Ankle Clin 2012; 17:687–706.

22. McCollum G, Myerson MS. Failure of the Agility™ total ankle replacement system and the salvage options. Clin Podiatr Med Surg 2013;30:207–23.

23. Ketz J, Myerson M, Sanders R. The salvage of complex hindfoot problems with use of a custom talar total ankle prosthesis. J Bone Joint Surg Am 2012;94:1194–200.

24. Myerson MS, Christensen JC, Steck JK, et al. Roundtable discussion: avascular necrosis of the foot and ankle. Foot Ankle Spec 2012;5:128–36.

25. Donnenwerth M, Roukis TS. Tibio-talo-calcaneal arthrodesis with retrograde intramedullary compression nail fixation for salvage of failed total ankle replacement: a systematic review. Clin Podiatr Med Surg 2013;30:199–206.

26. Henricson A, Rydholm U. Use of a trabecular metal implant in ankle arthrodesis after failed total ankle replacement. Acta Orthop 2010;81:745–7.

27. Horisberger M, Paul J, Wiewiorski M, et al. Commercially available trabecular metal ankle interpositional spacer for tibiotalocalcaneal arthrodesis secondary to severe bone loss of the ankle. J Foot Ankle Surg 2014;53:383–7.

Index

Note: Page numbers of article titles are in **boldface.**

A

Achilles tendon, lengthening of, for ankle equinus, 543–550
Agility systems
    complications of, arthroscopy for, 497
    failure of, salvage of, **609–616**
    learning curve for, 473–482
    replacement of
        complications of, **569–593**
        with Salto Talaris XT Revision Prosthesis, 552–567
    survival of, 483–494
Ankle equinus, correction of, during total ankle replacement, **543–550**
Ankle Evolutive System
    complications of, arthroscopy for, 498
    learning curve for, 473–482
    survival of, 483–494
Ankle replacement. *See* Total ankle replacement.
Anterior ankle arthroscopy, 499–501
Anterior gutter procedures, 498
Anteromedial pain syndrome, 498
AOA National Joint Replacement Registry, survival data from, 483–494
Arthroscopy and endoscopy, for complications, **495–508**
    far away from prosthesis, 505–506
    overview of, 496–497
    with close proximity to articular components, 497–503
    with close proximity to nonarticular components, 503–505

B

Bologna-Oxford system, survival of, 483–494
Bone, abnormal growth of, **509–516**
Bone cysts, arthroscopy for, 503–505
Bone graft
    for bone cysts, 504–505
    for failed INBONE device, 601–602
Broström-Gould lateral ankle stabilization, modified, for varus and valgus malalignment, 521–522, 527
Buechel-Pappas system
    complications of, arthroscopy for, 498
    learning curve for, 473–482
    survival of, 483–494

Clin Podiatr Med Surg 32 (2015) 617–622
http://dx.doi.org/10.1016/S0891-8422(15)00081-6
0891-8422/15/$ – see front matter © 2015 Elsevier Inc. All rights reserved.
podiatric.theclinics.com

United States Postal Service

Statement of Ownership, Management, and Circulation
(All Periodicals Publications Except Requestor Publications)

1. Publication Title	2. Publication Number	3. Filing Date
Clinics in Podiatric Medicine and Surgery	0 0 0 - 7 7 0 7	9/18/15

4. Issue Frequency	5. Number of Issues Published Annually	6. Annual Subscription Price
Jan, Apr, Jul, Oct	4	$305.00

7. Complete Mailing Address of Known Office of Publication (Not printer) (Street, city, county, state, and ZIP+4®)

Elsevier Inc.
360 Park Avenue South
New York, NY 10010-1710

Contact Person
Stephen R. Bushing
Telephone (Include area code)
215-239-3688

8. Complete Mailing Address of Headquarters or General Business Office of Publisher (Not printer)

Elsevier Inc., 360 Park Avenue South, New York, NY 10010-1710

9. Full Names and Complete Mailing Addresses of Publisher, Editor, and Managing Editor (Do not leave blank)

Publisher (Name and complete mailing address)

Linda Belfus, Elsevier Inc., 1600 John F. Kennedy Blvd., Ste. 1800, Philadelphia, PA 19103-2899

Editor (Name and complete mailing address)

Jennifer Flynn-Briggs, Elsevier, Inc., 1600 John F. Kennedy Blvd. Suite 1800, Philadelphia, PA 19103-2899

Managing Editor (Name and complete mailing address)

Adrianne Brigido, Elsevier, Inc., 1600 John F. Kennedy Blvd. Suite 1800, Philadelphia, PA 19103-2899

10. Owner (Do not leave blank. If the publication is owned by a corporation, give the name and address of the corporation immediately followed by the names and addresses of all stockholders owning or holding 1 percent or more of the total amount of stock. If not owned by a corporation, give the names and addresses of the individual owners. If owned by a partnership or other unincorporated firm, give its name and address as well as those of each individual owner. If the publication is published by a nonprofit organization, give its name and address.)

Full Name	Complete Mailing Address
Wholly owned subsidiary of	1600 John F. Kennedy Blvd, Ste. 1800
Reed/Elsevier, US holdings	Philadelphia, PA 19103-2899

11. Known Bondholders, Mortgagees, and Other Security Holders Owning or Holding 1 Percent or More of Total Amount of Bonds, Mortgages, or Other Securities. If none, check box ▸ ☐ None

Full Name	Complete Mailing Address
N/A	

12. Tax Status (For completion by nonprofit organizations authorized to mail at nonprofit rates) (Check one)
The purpose, function, and nonprofit status of this organization and the exempt status for federal income tax purposes:
☐ Has Not Changed During Preceding 12 Months
☐ Has Changed During Preceding 12 Months (Publisher must submit explanation of change with this statement)

13. Publication Title	14. Issue Date for Circulation Data Below
Clinics in Podiatric Medicine & Surgery	July 2015

PS Form 3526, July 2014 (Page 1 of 3 (Instructions Page 3)) PSN 7530-01-000-9931 PRIVACY NOTICE: See our Privacy policy in www.usps.com

---

15. Extent and Nature of Circulation			Average No. Copies Each Issue During Preceding 12 Months	No. Copies of Single Issue Published Nearest to Filing Date
a. Total Number of Copies (Net press run)			445	372
b. Legitimate Paid and Or Requested Distribution (By Mail and Outside the Mail)	(1)	Mailed Outside County Paid/Requested Mail Subscriptions stated on PS Form 3541. (Include paid distribution above nominal rate, advertiser's proof copies and exchange copies)	254	227
	(2)	Mailed In-County Paid/Requested Mail Subscriptions stated on PS Form 3541. (Include paid distribution above nominal rate, advertiser's proof copies and exchange copies)		
	(3)	Paid Distribution Outside the Mails Including Sales Through Dealers And Carriers, Street Vendors, Counter Sales, and Other Paid Distribution Outside USPS®	26	27
	(4)	Paid Distribution by Other Classes of Mail Through the USPS (e.g. First-Class Mail®)		
c. Total Paid and/or Requested Circulation (Sum of 15b (1), (2), (3), and (4)) ▸			280	254
d. Free or Nominal Rate Distribution (By Mail and Outside the Mail)	(1)	Free or Nominal Rate Outside-County Copies included on PS Form 3541	81	74
	(2)	Free or Nominal Rate In-County Copies Included on PS Form 3541		
	(3)	Free or Nominal Rate Copies mailed at Other classes Through the USPS (e.g. First-Class Mail®)		
	(4)	Free or Nominal Rate Distribution Outside the Mail (Carriers or Other means)		
e. Total Nonrequested Distribution (Sum of 15d (1), (2), (3) and (4)) ▸			81	74
f. Total Distribution (Sum of 15c and 15e) ▸			361	328
g. Copies not Distributed (See instructions to publishers #4 (page #3)) ▸			84	44
h. Total (Sum of 15f and g) ▸			445	372
i. Percent Paid and/or Requested Circulation (15c divided by 15f times 100) ▸			77.56%	77.44%

* If you are claiming electronic copies go to line 16 on page 3. If you are not claiming Electronic copies, skip to line 17 on page 3.

16. Electronic Copy Circulation		Average No. Copies Each Issue During Preceding 12 Months	No. Copies of Single Issue Published Nearest to Filing Date
a. Paid Electronic Copies ▸			
b. Total paid Print Copies (Line 15c) + Paid Electronic copies (Line 16a) ▸			
c. Total Print Distribution (Line 15f) + Paid Electronic Copies (Line 16a) ▸			
d. Percent Paid (Both Print & Electronic copies) (16b divided by 16c X 100) ▸			

☐ I certify that 50% of all my distributed copies (electronic and print) are paid above a nominal price

17. Publication of Statement of Ownership
If the publication is a general publication, publication of this statement is required. Will be printed in the **October 2015** issue of this publication.

18. Signature and Title of Editor, Publisher, Business Manager, or Owner	Date
Stephen R. Bushing	September 18, 2015
Stephen R. Bushing – Inventory Distribution Coordinator	

I certify that all information furnished on this form is true and complete. I understand that anyone who furnishes false or misleading information on this form or who omits material or information requested on the form may be subject to criminal sanctions (including fines and imprisonment) and/or civil sanctions (including civil penalties).

PS Form 3526, July 2014 (Page 3 of 3)

Printed and bound by CPI Group (UK) Ltd, Croydon, CR0 4YY

07/10/2024

01040500-0012